Compact Clinical Guide to

ARRHYTHMIA AND 12-LEAD
EKG INTERPRETATION

Sandra Goldsworthy, PhD, MSc, RN, CNCC(C), CMSN(C), is a recognized critical care expert, researcher, and author. She is the author or editor of six books, including *Stimulation Simplified: A Practical Guide for Nurse Educators, Simulation Simplified: Student Lab Manual for Critical Care Nursing,* and *The Compact Clinical Guide for Mechanical Ventilation.* She is an associate professor in the faculty of nursing at the University of Calgary, where she holds a research professorship in simulation education. She holds two national Canadian Nurses Association credentials in critical care and medical–surgical nursing. She is a member of a number of national and international committees, including serving on the board of directors for the World Federation of Critical Care Nurses Association. Her research focus is on simulation and transfer of learning, job readiness, and transition of new graduates into critical care, and she has conducted and published research involving the use of simulation and technology in nursing education. Her recent publications and national and international presentations have concentrated on critical care nurse retention, critical care nurse work environments, and the use of simulation to build confidence and competence among nurses.

Compact Clinical Guide to

ARRHYTHMIA AND 12-LEAD EKG INTERPRETATION

Foundations of Practice for Critical Care Nurses

Sandra Goldsworthy, PhD, MSc, RN, CNCC(C), CMSN(C)

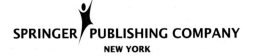

SPRINGER PUBLISHING COMPANY
NEW YORK

Springer Publishing Company, LLC
11 West 42nd Street
New York, NY 10036
www.springerpub.com

Acquisitions Editor: Elizabeth Nieginski
Composition: diacriTech

ISBN: 978-0-8261-9846-4
e-book ISBN: 978-0-8261-9847-1
PowerPoint ISBN: 978-0-8261-9629-3

Student supplements are available from www.springerpub.com/goldsworthy

16   17   18   19   /   5   4   3   2   1

The author and the publisher of this Work have made every effort to use sources believed to be reliable to provide information that is accurate and compatible with the standards generally accepted at the time of publication. Because medical science is continually advancing, our knowledge base continues to expand. Therefore, as new information becomes available, changes in procedures become necessary. We recommend that the reader always consult current research and specific institutional policies before performing any clinical procedure. The author and publisher shall not be liable for any special, consequential, or exemplary damages resulting, in whole or in part, from the readers' use of, or reliance on, the information contained in this book. The publisher has no responsibility for the persistence or accuracy of URLs for external or third-party Internet websites referred to in this publication and does not guarantee that any content on such websites is, or will remain, accurate or appropriate.

Library of Congress Cataloging-in-Publication Data

Names: Goldsworthy, Sandra, 1961- author.
Title: Compact clinical guide to arrhythmia and 12-lead ekg interpretation: foundations of
    practice for critical care nurses / Sandra Goldsworthy, PhD, RN, MSc, CNCC(C), CMSN(C).
Description: New York, NY : Springer Publishing Company, LLC, [2016] |
    Includes bibliographical references and index.
Identifiers: LCCN 2016014653| ISBN 9780826198464 | ISBN 9780826198471 (ebook)
Subjects: LCSH: Arrhythmia—Diagnosis. | Electrocardiography—Interpretation.
    | Heart—Electric properties.
Classification: LCC RC685.A65 G65 2016 | DDC 616.1/28—dc23 LC record available at
https://lccn.loc.gov/2016014653

Printed in the United States of America by Gasch Printing.

I dedicate this book to all the wonderful nursing students whom I have had the privilege to teach over the past 28 years. It has truly enriched my life and it has been a pleasure.

Contents

Preface

One of the foundational competencies required of critical care nurses is the ability to interpret cardiac rhythms systematically. Failure to recognize and respond to dangerous arrhythmias could lead to serious life-threatening consequences for the patient.

Through my teaching of cardiac arrhythmia courses and advanced cardiac life support (ACLS) to nurses and other health professionals over the past three decades, I have developed strategies to help bedside practitioners rapidly interpret abnormal cardiac rhythms and to determine how to prioritize interventions quickly. The amount of information on this topic can be overwhelming, and there are many different types of education available on the market about arrhythmia/12-lead EKGs. The goal of this text is to be user friendly by striking a balance between cue cards or a basic overview and text-dense lengthy explanations. This text is aimed at being a bedside reference small enough to carry in a nurse's pocket, yet still containing enough detail to provide the nurse with critical information needed at the point of care.

The text begins with a brief overview of the anatomy and physiology related to the heart and its conduction system. The chapters that follow align with specific pacemaker sites related to arrhythmias (i.e., sinus, atrial, junctional, ventricular, atrioventricular [AV] heart blocks, and paced rhythms). In addition, an introduction to 12-lead EKGs is presented with content related to myocardial infarction.

The *Compact Clinical Guide to Arrhythmia and 12-Lead EKG Interpretation: Foundations of Practice for Critical Care Nurses* specifically includes a systematic approach to basic arrhythmia interpretation, examples, and explanations of all of the basic sinus, atrial, ventricular, and AV heart block arrhythmias; a systematic approach to 12-lead EKG interpretation; and a systematic approach to pacemaker rhythm interpretation and malfunction. To further consolidate your learning, each chapter ends with practice questions and a case study you can use to test yourself. **Associated electronic resources that accompany this text are cue cards of systematic approaches for arrhythmia, 12-lead EKG, and pacemaker interpretation provided as a PowerPoint presentation that can be accessed from www.springerpub.com/goldsworthy.** The most current guidelines are incorporated into this text, including the newest *2015 American Heart Association Guidelines for Cardiac and Emergency Care.*

Most important, I hope you will benefit from the clinical tips integrated into each chapter. Because we do not see all rhythms regularly in clinical practice, and some are very rare, you may find it helpful to review the content in this text at regular intervals.

I hope you will find this resource helpful as you care for critically ill patients in your practice. It has been a pleasure creating it!

Sandra Goldsworthy

Acknowledgments

I would like to acknowledge the team at Springer Publishing Company, especially executive editor extraordinaire, Elizabeth Nieginski, who is always a pleasure to work with and a true and gracious professional. I appreciate all of their efforts in bringing this book to fruition. I would also like to acknowledge the contribution of Wendy Preiano, nursing professor at Georgian College, for writing the first chapter of the book. Her efforts are greatly appreciated.

1

Basic Anatomy and Physiology: Highlights

Wendy Preiano

OBJECTIVES

By reading and studying this chapter, the learner will be able to:

1. Describe the heart's basic function, size, shape, and location
2. Identify and explain the four heart chambers, the three layers of the heart, and the four heart valves
3. Understand blow flow and coronary circulation
4. Explain cardiac conduction, including the four common characteristics of heart cells, three phases of normal electrical activity of the heart (polarization, depolarization, and repolarization), and the conduction pathways
5. Describe the heart's blood pressure (BP), cardiac output (CO), and associated terms

Every day the average heart and cardiac system pumps about 1,200 L (1,900 gallons) through the body and beats about 100,000 times. The primary function of the heart and cardiac system is circulation; together with the lungs, the cardiac system delivers oxygen-rich (oxygenated) blood and nutrients to the body, tissues, and organs. Precise and complex regulatory mechanisms work collaboratively to balance metabolic demands of cardiac tissue and cardiac output (CO). As with all the bodily organs and systems, a clear and concise understanding of anatomy and physiology directly correlates to how and where systems can fail.

HEART SIZE, SHAPE, AND LOCATION

The heart is a hollow and strong double-sided muscular pump located in the mediastinum (between and in front of the lungs, in front of the spinal column, just above the diaphragm, with its bulk behind the sternum). The size of a person's closed fist, the heart tilts slightly lateral left with about two thirds to the left of the midline of the sternum and about one third to the right of the midline of the sternum. As such, the right ventricle has the largest anterior surface area. Its weight and size are all relative to the person's age, size, physical condition, and heart health.

Different from other organs, the heart is upside down with its broader top-end base found between the second intercostal space on the right and left sternal borders. The apex, which tapers to a rounded end, is tilted down and slightly left. During each heartbeat, the apex strikes against the chest wall, causing a thrust or **point of maximal impulse (PMI)**, which when palpated, is felt at the left midclavicular area in the fifth or sixth intercostal space. The PMI is also termed the *apical pulse.*

The **cardiac cycle** refers to repetitive pumping of the heart that includes all parts of the heart working synchronistically to create blood flow through the heart and the body. It depends on both the heart's mechanical ability to contract and its conduction system.

THE HEART'S CHAMBERS

The heart houses four separate hollow chambers—two upper atria and two lower ventricles, which are separated by a muscular septum.

The Atria	*The Septum*	*The Ventricles*
The top, receiving chambers are the thin-walled atria; they *collect blood coming from the body and lungs back to the heart.* Each atrium contracts at the same time to deliver blood to the lower ventricles.	The septum separates the left and right sides of the heart. *The interatrial septum separates the atria* and the *interventricular septum separates the ventricles.*	Through strong and rhythmic contractions, *the* ventricles *pump blood away from the heart* to the body and lungs.

THE LAYERS OF THE HEART

The heart has many layers, each of which has unique characteristics that work collaboratively to function efficiently. From the outermost to innermost layer, each part has unique and dynamic functions, which ensure that circulation is fluid and smooth, allowing for changes in body temperature, stress, and illness.

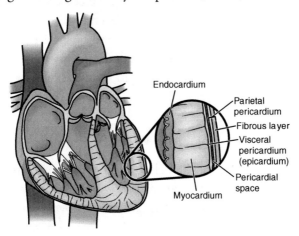

The **outer pericardium** (literally meaning "around the heart") is the tightly fitted double-layered sac that swaddles the heart. The tough parietal pericardium attaches to the sternum and the diaphragm. About 10 to 30 mL of serous fluid is located between the visceral and parietal pericardial layers; this pericardial fluid lubricates and prevents friction with each cardiac contraction. The thin space that contains the pericardial fluid is known as the **pericardial space.** The **epicardium** or visceral pericardium is the outer protective layer of he heart that is composed primarily of mesothelium, which is a simple squamous tissue. This area is where the coronary arteries are innervated.

The next and largest layer is the strong, middle muscle layer, the **myocardium**. Cardiac muscle is striated and unique to the heart, as it produces the heart's contraction, or the heartbeat that is measured. Each individual muscle cell is called a **cardiac myocyte** and different ones have both the ability to pump and transmit an electrical impulse. Myocardial tissue is thinnest in the atria and thickest in the ventricles, with the thickest layer on the left ventricle, as this area must be the strongest, because it works to pump blood to all parts of the body.

The innermost layer of tissue lining the heart is the **endocardium**, which is continuous with the endothelial layer found throughout the body (in arteries, veins, and capillaries), the heart's chambers, valves, chordae tendineae, and papillary muscles. These squamous epithelial cells are smooth to allow ease of flow of blood and to decrease the chance of clots.

HEART VALVES

Heart valves are smooth, delicate, supple extensions of the endocardium that control the direction of blood flow, preventing backflow. The main valves are the atrioventricular (AV) and semilunar (SL) valves.

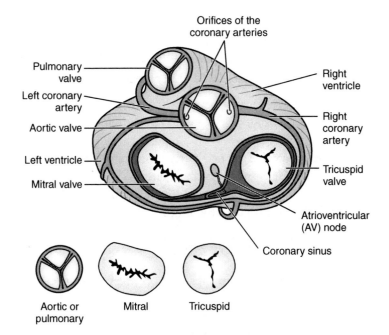

The **AV valves** are, as the name suggests, located between the atria and ventricles and open passively during diastole, when atrial pressure in blood is greater than ventricular pressure. They are attached to papillary muscles by tough chordae tendineae, which make sure valves do not turn inside out. To control constant tension on delicate valve leaflets, papillary muscles contract simultaneously with the ventricles.

■ The **tricuspid valve** has three cusps and it lies between the right atrium and the right ventricle. Open, oxygen-poor blood flows through the right atrium into the right ventricle; closed, it forces contraction of the right ventricle to push blood through the SL valve into the pulmonary artery.

■ The **bicuspid or mitral valve** has two cusps and it lies between the left atrium and ventricle. It opens to permit oxygen-rich blood to flow from the right atrium to the right ventricle.

SL valves are thicker then AV valves and open and close passively according to a pressure gradient, similar to AV valves. SL valves open when intraventricular pressure is greater than pulmonary and aortic pressure and close when the pressures reverse.

- The **aortic valve**, located between the left ventricle and aorta, opens to permit oxygen-rich blood to flow from the left ventricle to the rest of the body.
- The **pulmonic valve** sits on the right side of the heart between the right ventricle and pulmonary artery. During ventricular contraction it opens, permitting oxygen-poor blood to flow from the right ventricle to the lungs.

Helpful Tips

- Normal heart sounds are created when the heart valves shut, causing the chambers and major arteries to vibrate.
- The **first heart sound, S1** or "lub," is loudest at the apex and is the result of the closing of the AV valves.
- The **second heart sound, S2** or "dub," is loudest at the base and is the result of the closing of the SL valves.

BLOOD FLOW AND CORONARY CIRCULATION

The circulatory system is responsible for the flow of blood and nutrients in the entire body; coronary circulation is part of the circulatory system and it supplies blood specifically to the heart. Blood flow from the heart to the lungs and body are two separate but mutually supporting systems. Simultaneously, while the left ventricle pushes blood through the aorta, the right ventricle pushes blood through the pulmonary artery to the lungs. The heart is unique as it not only has two interdependent pumps, but also houses its own mini circulatory system to deliver and feed itself oxygen prior to any other body organs. It feeds itself first because as the heart continuously contracts and relaxes it requires its own blood supply.

Blood Flow

The body's circulatory system sends blood from the heart to the lungs, back to the heart and out to the body. The route of pulmonary and systemic circulation flows as follows:

- Right atrium receives venous blood from the inferior and superior venae cavae and the coronary sinus → blood passes through the tricuspid valve → right ventricle depolarizes/contracts to send blood out → pulmonic valve → pulmonary artery → onto the lungs (where blood becomes oxygenated) → left atrium by way of the pulmonary veins → mitral (bicuspid) valve → left ventricle depolarizes/contracts to push blood → aortic valve → aorta → systemic and coronary circulation

Helpful Tips

- **Systemic circulation:** the *left side of the heart's ability to deliver oxygen-rich blood to the tissues* via the arteries.
- **Pulmonary circulation:** the *right side of the heart's ability to receive oxygen-poor blood* back from the body from the veins and to pump it to and through the lungs.
- The thick septum divides the right and left sides of the heart into two separate yet synchronized pumps.
- Failure of either the right or left side of the heart, if not corrected, can lead to dysfunction of the other side.
- **Pulmonary arteries:** the only arteries in the body that house deoxygenated (oxygen-poor) blood.
- **Pulmonary veins:** the only veins in the body that carry (oxygen-rich) oxygenated blood.

Coronary Circulation

Coronary circulation involves the heart's blood supply, which includes coronary arteries and veins. The arteries branch off into smaller arterioles and then smaller capillaries where oxygen and nutrients are exchanged. After this, the blood moves to venules (smallest veins) and then back to bigger veins.

- Fresh *oxygen-rich blood (oxygenated) is mainly supplied by the right and left coronary arteries* that branch off the base of the aorta near the aortic valve.
- *Oxygen-poor blood (deoxygenated) is returned to the right atrium via the coronary veins* whose divisions run parallel to the coronary arteries.
- *Autoregulation of the coronary arteries*: a term denoting the ability of the coronary arteries to constantly adjust blood flow based on tissue demand. This is necessary for the heart's own perfusion.
- *Vasoconstriction* of the coronary arteries: decreased arterial vessel diameter caused by decreased metabolic activity or increased driving pressure.
- *Vasodilation* of the coronary arteries: increased vessel diameter caused by increased tissue metabolism or reduced driving pressure.

Coronary arteries that supply the heart muscle with oxygen:

- The left main coronary artery *descends into the left circumflex and left anterior descending (LAD) artery.* The LAD feeds the septum between the ventricles (intraventricular septum) and anterior (front and bottom) of the left ventricle. As its name suggests, the **circumflex artery** "curves" around the left ventricle, supplying the lateral wall (side and back) of the left ventricle and the left atrium.
- The **right coronary artery (RCA)** provides blood to the right atrium, right ventricle, bottom portion of the left ventricle, and back of the septum.

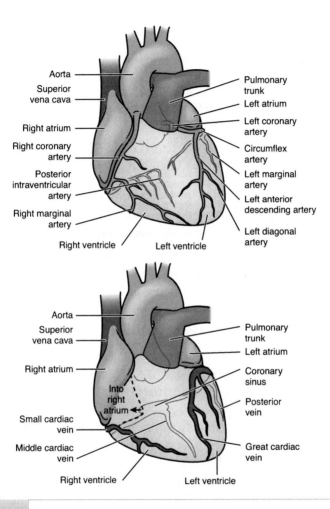

During diastole (relaxation) blood flows into the **coronary arteries.** Any impairment in diastole can impair filling of the heart's arteries (i.e., congestive heart failure, cardiomyopathy, pericarditis).

Housed within the myocardium, coronary arteries begin on the epicardial surface and end on the endocardial surface.

As a result of this anatomy, the earliest sign of myocyte ischemia (lack of oxygen) is ST depression on an EKG.

> *Clinical Pearls* The RCA supplies sections of the heart's conduction system, including the AV node and bundle of His. If there is an issue in this artery, serious cardiac conduction defects can occur as well as inferior or right ventricular myocardial infarctions with blockage of the RCA.

THE HEART'S INTRINSIC CONDUCTION SYSTEM AND THE HEART'S ELECTRICAL SYSTEM

The heart is unique as it is in charge of its own mini circulation and is able to respond to and generate an electrical impulse that creates the beating heart (contraction and relaxation). To do so, *heart cells are specialized pacemaker cells* that have four unique characteristics and that use the sodium–potassium pump to depolarize and repolarize and house an orderly pathway for electrical conduction.

Four electrical properties of specialized pacemaker cells are:

1. *Automaticity:* the heart's ability to spontaneously generate and initiate an electrical impulse. It is this property that allows the normal pacemaker cells (sinoatrial [SA] node) to spontaneously initiate its own impulse.
2. *Conduction:* the heart cells ability to transmit an impulse to neighboring cells along a set pathway.
3. *Contractility:* the ability of heart cells to receive and respond to an impulse by shortening fibers and thereby contract.
4. *Excitability:* the ability of the heart cells to react and respond to an electrical impulse.

- **Refractory period or refractory phase:** the resting period after stimulation. The refractory period is divided into two phases: absolute refractory period (or the period when the heart cannot accept another impulse) and the relative refractory period (when a stronger-than-normal impulse may cause depolarization). If an impulse arises during this relative refractory period, lethal arrhythmias can occur such as ventricular fibrillation. This is referred to as "R on T" phenomena and will be discussed further in Chapter 2.

Helpful Tips

The **cardiac cycle:** the process that fills and drains the heart's chambers.

The **conduction system:** the electrical system of the heart (that creates an action potential). It permits the cardiac cycle to rhythmically continue without interruption.

The **mechanical system:** the movement, the contraction, and the relaxation of the heart that is triggered by the conduction system.

Also, electrical activity must occur before there is mechanical activity. In the case of pulseless electrical activity (PEA), there is electrical activity but no subsequent mechanical activity. See Chapter 5 for common causes of PEA.

Clinical Pearls

If necrosis of myocardial tissue occurs (myocardial infarction), then the electrical and the mechanical properties of the heart are affected. The electrical impulse cannot travel through dead or necrotic tissue and must go around it, causing abnormalities in conduction and delays in conduction speed.

Sodium–Potassium Pump

Normal electrical activity of the heart has three phases with many signals that require potassium (K^+) and sodium (Na^+) ions. It is the electrical energy (action potential) created by the exchange of these ions that stimulates the heart to beat.

Phase One: **Polarization**. Cells are considered ready to receive an electrical impulse when the cell is negatively charged. (This reflects the normal ratio of the sodium–potassium pump; K^+ on the inside of the cell and Na^+ on the outside of the cell.)

Phase Two: **Depolarization** (which causes *contraction*). Here, the heart cells transmit an electrical spark when Na^+ moves into the cell and K^+ moves out of the cell. As the cell is positively charged, it will create a contraction.

Helpful Tips

Depolarization is the electrical event and contraction is the mechanical event.

Phase Three: **Repolarization**. Cells in this recovery stage send K^+ inside the cell and Na^+ outside to return the cell to a balanced state.

Clinical Pearls

PEA: electrical activity on the cardiac monitor and absence of a pulse.

Depolarization and the EKG:

- **P wave: atrial depolarization**. As the atria are depolarized and stimulated a P wave is seen.
- **QRS complex: ventricular depolarization.** As the ventricles depolarize a QRS complex is seen.

Repolarization and the EKG:

- **ST segment and T wave: ventricular repolarization.** Ventricles begin to recover and restore their electrical charge.

Calcium (Ca^{++}) also stimulates a contraction in the myocardium.

- Some drugs, such as calcium channel blockers (e.g., verapamil and diltiazem), can decrease the rate that Ca^{++} enters the cells, thereby slowing contractions.

THE NORMAL INTRINSIC CONDUCTION PATHWAY— HOW ELECTRICAL IMPULSES FLOW THROUGH THE HEART

During a heartbeat, the normal conduction pathway follows a sequential order. The route of electrical impulse is as follows:

SA node → travels through intra-arterial and internodal pathways → AV node → bundle of His → left and right bundle branches (BBs) → ends in the Purkinje fibers after which time the ventricles contract.

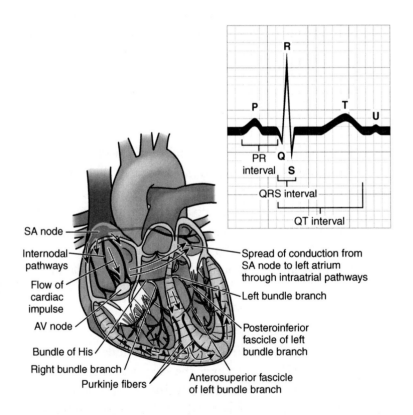

The SA Node

The **SA node** is considered the heart's natural pacemaker cell; it usually initiates the conduction pathway and sets the pace of the heart. A cluster of specialized nerve fibers, the SA node is located in the right atrium, close to the superior vena cava; it typically fires at a rate of 60 to 100 times per minute (the average heartbeat or **normal sinus rhythm [NSR]**). Atrial contraction (depolarization) occurs as the SA node transmits an electrical impulse through both the right and left atria, which travels through the intra-arterial pathway. This intrinsic pathway is a fibrous skeleton that divides the atrial and ventricular myocardium so that electrical conduction only affects the atria.

The **internodal pathway** links the SA node to the AV node and is located in the walls of the atria. At this point, both the SA node and the internodal pathway repolarize.

The AV Node

The **AV node** is located low in the septal wall of the right atrium and is considered the *resistor node* as it slows down the electrical impulse between the atria and ventricles. This is very important so that the ventricles have time to fill with blood prior to ventricular contraction. The AV node usually transmits at a rate of 40 to 60 impulses per minute and can become the secondary pacemaker should the initial SA node fail to function.

Bundle of His and BBs

Modified muscle fibers found below the AV node are known as the **bundle of His**. They carry the electrical impulse to the right and left **BBs.** The right and left BBs divide and supply the right and left sides of the heart and fire the electrical impulse to the Purkinje fibers.

Purkinje Fibers

The **Purkinjes** are the distal portions of the BBs that extend from the endocardium into the muscular ventricular wall to conduct an electrical impulse that initiates contraction of the heart muscle. Should both the SA and AV node fail to conduct an electrical impulse, the ventricles can initiate and transmit their own electrical impulse, generally at a much slower rate of 20 to 40 per minute.

Important Points to Remember

1. The heart's **cardiac conduction system** generates and initiates depolarization then contraction.
2. **Electrical impulses,** which are action potentials, follow a sequential **conduction pathway** that results in the heart's contraction.
3. An **EKG** records the heart's electrical activity (not the heart's pumping action).
4. **Cardiac dysrhythmias** are altered electrical stimulation of the heart that disturb the synchronized pathway of contractions and the heart's efficiency. These dysrhythmias may be benign or deadly and the causes vary, including fever, stress, exercise, hypoxia, caffeine, drugs, or many cardiac, lung, or metabolic states.
5. An **ectopic beat** is any pacemaker cell that initiates and generates an electrical impulse outside of the SA node (the normal pacemaker). This can result in a dysrhythmia (examples of ectopic pacemakers that can "take over" as a result of factors such as ischemia are: the atria, the AV node, the ventricles). When the atria take over as pacemaker for the heart, rhythms such as atrial flutter can occur. When the AV node becomes

---

(continued)

(continued)

> the pacemaker of the heart, junctional rhythms result. Finally, when the ventricle takes over as the pacemaker of the heart, an altered rhythm, such as idioventricular rhythm, can be seen. These rhythms will be discussed in the next few chapters of this text.
>
> **6.** An **escape rhythm** is a rhythm that arises from the AV node or ventricles (not the SA node). Although this is protective, any rate other than the SA node is too slow to meet the body's oxygen demands. Often, an artificial pacemaker may be required to maintain CO.

Clinical Pearls

AV blocks: caused by depolarization and repolarization, which are slower in the AV node, making this region more susceptible to conduction blocks

Junctional arrhythmias: irregular cardiac rhythms that start near or within the AV node

Supraventricular arrhythmias: abnormal cardiac rhythms that develop above the bundle of His or stimulate the ventricles through an accessory pathway (usually above the ventricles)

Ventricular arrhythmias: abnormal cardiac rhythms that initiate below the bundle of His

---

BP AND CO

Depolarization generates functional movement of the muscular layer (a contraction) of the heart. **Systole** is the strong muscular heart contraction that ejects blood from the ventricles. **Diastole** is the relaxation phase that allows for blood to fill the ventricles. Arterial pressures rise during systole and fall in diastole. **BP** is the measurement of pressure exerted by blood against the arterial walls. Simply put, *BP is systole/diastole.* BP is influenced by both baroreceptors and chemoreceptors.

■ **Baroreceptors** are specialized nerve tissue located in the internal carotid arteries and the receptors at the base of the aortic arch that detects changes in BP. When stimulated they elicit a response in the autonomic nervous system.

■ **Chemoreceptors** are sensory receptors located in the carotid body and aortic arch that detect changes in the concentration of pH, oxygen, and carbon dioxide.

CO is the amount of blood pumped by each ventricle in 1 minute. CO equals stroke volume (SV; the amount of blood ejected from the ventricle with each heartbeat) × heart rate (HR).

CO can be affected by anything that changes SV or HR. HR is primarily affected by the autonomic nervous system (ANS) and SV is affected by preload and afterload.

■ **Preload:** *degree of ventricular stretch* based on the volume of blood coming into the ventricle. According the Frank–Starling law, the more the myocardium is stretched, the greater the force of contraction.

■ **Afterload:** *the "squeeze"; the resistance the ventricle must overcome to pump blood to the body.* Afterload is sometime referred to as *systemic vascular resistance.* Afterload increases with hypertension and aortic stenosis. There is right-sided afterload (the resistance the heart has to overcome to pump to the lungs—should be low pressure and left-sided afterload (the amount of resistance the heart has to overcome to pump blood out to the body).

The Autonomic Nervous System

Based on the body's and heart's changing demands, the cardiac system needs to adjust and the ANS helps to respond to these adjustments. The SA and the AV nodes are innervated within the two parts of the ANS, which are the sympathetic nervous system (SNS) and the parasympathetic nervous system (PNS).

Important Points to Remember

1. **SNS** (the "fight or flight" response—speeds everything up). Stimulation of the sympathetic system increases HR, speed of AV node conduction, and the power of contractions in both the atria and ventricles. It is innervated by beta-adrenergic receptors that accept norepinephrine and epinephrine.
2. **PNS** ("the brakes"—slows everything down). This system opposes the SNS; stimulation of the parasympathetic system slows HR and conduction through the AV node. This system is innervated by the vagus nerve. Vagal nerve stimulation causes a decrease in all of the following: the rate of SA node firing, impulse conduction of the AV node, and force of contraction.

Clinical Pearls

Inotropes: *factors affecting contractility*

- Positive inotropic drugs increase the heart's contractility such as digitalis, dobutamine
- Negative inotropic drugs decrease the heart's contractility such as beta blockers and calcium channel blockers

Chronotropes: *factors that affect change in the HR*

- Positive chronotropes increase HR such as adrenaline
- Negative chronotropes decrease HR such as digoxin

Dromotropes: *factors that affect speed of conduction*

- Positive dromotropes: increase in AV conduction such as phenytoin
- Negative dromotropes: decrease in AV conduction such as verapamil

EXERCISES

Test Yourself!

1. What factors impact SV?
2. What does the term *inotropic* mean?
3. What do the following EKG waveforms represent:
   a. P wave
   b. QRS
   c. T wave
   d. QT interval
4. Depolarization is considered to lead to the phase of:
   a. Contraction
   b. Recovery
   c. Readiness
   d. Transportation
5. The heart's ability to spontaneously generate and initiate an electrical impulse is termed:
   a. Automaticity
   b. Conductivity
   c. Contractility
   d. Excitability
6. Outline the normal intrinsic conduction pathway within the heart.

(See answers for Chapter 1 in the "Answers" chapter.)

RESOURCES

Atwood, S., Stanton, C., & Storey-Davenport, J. (2011). *Basic cardiac dysrhythmias* (4th ed.). St. Louis, MO: Elsevier.

Barry, M., Goldsworthy, S., Lok, J., & Tyreman, J. (Eds.). (in press). *Medical-surgical nursing in Canada: Assessment and management of clinical problems* (4th Canadian ed.). Toronto, ON: Elsevier Mosby.

Copstead, L., & Banasik, J. (2013). *Pathophysiology* (5th ed.). St. Louis, MO: Elsevier Saunders.

2

Arrhythmias: Sinus and Atrial

SINUS RHYTHMS

In this chapter, sinus and atrial rhythms are discussed. Specifically, the following rhythms are presented: normal sinus rhythm, sinus bradycardia, sinus tachycardia, sinus arrhythmia, and sinus arrest/block. The atrial rhythms discussed are premature atrial contractions (PACs), atrial fibrillation, atrial flutter, and supraventricular tachycardia (SVT). Unique characteristics, causes, treatment, and tips for interpretation are provided. In addition, practice examples, "test yourself" questions, and an integrated case study are provided at the end of the chapter to help you retain the need-to-know information and build your confidence in interpreting arrhythmias.

Helpful Tips

Unique characteristics of each rhythm that help differentiate it from others are in **boldface**.

Normal Sinus Rhythm (aka the "Benchmark" Rhythm)

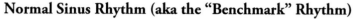

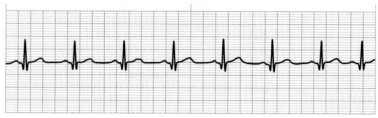

Figure 2.1 ▦ Normal sinus rhythm.

Unique Characteristics

Rhythm	Regular
Rate	60–100 beats/minute
P waves	Present, upright, symmetrical, one before every QRS
PRi (PR interval)	0.12–0.20 seconds
QRS	0.06–0.10 seconds

Normal sinus rhythm is considered to be the hemodynamically "perfect" or benchmark rhythm. We compare all other rhythms to this baseline. Normal sinus rhythm can only have these characteristics, as listed in the previous grid. If the rhythm has these characteristics, but perhaps has an elevated ST segment, we then refer to it as sinus rhythm with an elevated ST segment. It is not truly "normal" sinus rhythm unless it has the unique characteristics as listed in the previous grid.

Causes

This rhythm is normal and does not have underlying pathology.

Treatment

No treatment is required for normal sinus rhythm.

Tips for Interpretation

Remember, if the rhythm does not have all of the characteristics listed earlier, then *it is not* normal sinus rhythm. Be careful to actually measure regularity with this rhythm because it can closely mimic other rhythms such as sinus arrhythmia. Never fall into the trap of "estimating" rhythms with the naked eye, make sure to *always use the systematic approach.*

Clinical Pearls

How to Recognize Stable Versus Unstable

What defines *unstable*?

■ Vital organ function is acutely impaired or cardiac arrest is imminent
  ✓ Respiratory failure
  ✓ Profound hypotension
  ✓ Severe hypoxemia
  ✓ Ischemic chest pain
  ✓ Acute heart failure
  ✓ Other signs of shock
  ✓ Altered mental status
■ Treatment is required, immediately, without delay for unstable rhythms

What defines *stable*?

■ The arrhythmia is causing symptoms but the patient is stable and there is time to consider pharmacological interventions.
    The patient may exhibit such symptoms as:
  ✓ Palpitations
  ✓ Lightheadedness
  ✓ dyspnea
(American Heart Association [AHA], 2015)

Sinus Bradycardia

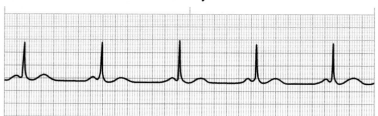

Figure 2.2 ■ Sinus bradycardia.

Unique Characteristics

Rhythm	Regular
Rate	**40–60 beats/minute (heart rate may be lower than 40 beats/minute)**
P waves	Upright, symmetrical, one before every QRS
PRi	0.12–0.20 seconds
QRS	0.06–0.10 seconds

Causes

There are a number of causes of sinus bradycardia but the most common include *parasympathetic (vagal) stimulation* (e.g., *vomiting*, endotracheal *suctioning*, and *carotid sinus pressure*) and hypoxemia. Carotid sinus pressure can be inadvertently caused by a shirt collar that is too tight or a tie that is too snug. Carotid sinus pressure (i.e., carotid sinus massage) can also be intentionally applied by experienced medical personnel in the instance of rapid SVTs to slow the heart rate. Sinus bradycardia can also occur in *myocardial infarctions* (MIs) especially those involving the *inferior or the posterior portions* of the heart. It is important to remember that sinus bradycardia *can be normal* and can occur *while sleeping* or in conditioned *athlete's hearts*, which are exceedingly efficient.

Treatment

Because sinus bradycardia can be a normal aberration, it is *only treated if the patient is unstable or symptomatic*. The first-line drug of choice for symptomatic sinus bradycardia is atropine. *Atropine* is a vagolytic drug that "lyses" or "breaks" the effect of the parasympathetic nervous system to increase the heart rate. The dosage is 0.5 mg every 3 to 5 minutes (to a maximum of 3 mg) and it is administered via intravenous (IV) push (AHA, 2010). Should the patient become unstable, *transcutaneous pacing* or a vasopressor infusion, such as *dopamine* or *epinephrine*, is the treatment of choice (AHA, 2010). The recommended dosage for dopamine is 2 to 10 mcg/kg/minute and the dosage for epinephrine is 2 to 10 mcg/minute. Pacemakers and paced rhythms will be discussed further in Chapter 5.

Tips for Interpretation

Sinus bradycardia looks very similar to normal sinus rhythm with one exception: *the rate is slower*.

Sinus Tachycardia

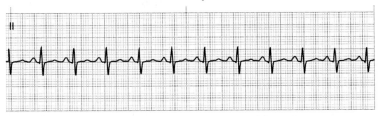

Figure 2.3 ■ Sinus tachycardia.

Unique Characteristics

Rhythm	Regular
Rate	**100–150 beats/minute (rate may be faster than 150 beats/minute)**
P waves	Upright, symmetrical, one before every QRS
PRi	0.12–0.20 seconds
QRS	0.06–0.10 seconds

Causes

The most common cause of sinus tachycardia is *sympathetic stimulation* or hypoxia. The most frequent triggers of this rhythm are exercise, *pain*, *fever*, and *anxiety*. There can also be more ominous causes such as shock, MI, heart failure, infection, hyperthyroidism, caffeine, medications (e.g., epinephrine, dopamine), nicotine, and cocaine.

Treatment

The recommended treatment for sinus tachycardia is to *treat the underlying cause*. Depending on the cause of this rhythm, the treatments could include administration of fluid and an analgesic, removal of medications causing the rhythm, and so on.

Tips for Interpretation

Sinus tachycardia looks very similar to normal sinus rhythm with one exception: the rate is faster.

Sinus Arrhythmia

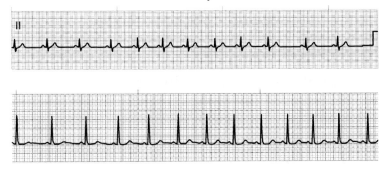

Figure 2.4 ■ Examples of sinus arrhythmia.

Unique Characteristics

Rhythm	Irregular
Rate	60–100 beats/minute
P waves	Upright, symmetrical, one before every QRS
PRi	0.12–0.20 seconds
QRS	0.06–0.10 seconds

Causes

This rhythm can be caused by *changes in intrathoracic pressure,* hence the changes in rate, with some faster beats and other periods with slower beats corresponding to inspiration and expiration, respectively. Sinus arrhythmia can also be seen in healthy hearts, especially in *children or young adults* (< 30 years of age). Other causes include *inferior MI, increased intracranial pressure,* and *medications* (e.g., digoxin or morphine).

Treatment

No treatment is required for this benign rhythm.

Tips for Interpretation

Sinus arrhythmia looks very similar to normal sinus rhythm with one exception: *The rhythm is irregular.* In fact, you will notice the rhythm can often have a pattern of speeding up and slowing down (sometimes in relation to inspiration and expiration), therefore you will see that part of the rhythm has a quicker pace and then it slows and the process repeats itself.

Sinus Arrest

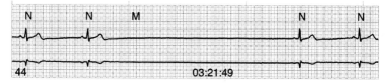

Figure 2.5 ■ Sinus arrest.

Unique Characteristics

Rhythm	Irregular (caused by missed beat or "pause")
Rate	Underlying rhythm usually 60–100 beats/minute
P waves	Present, upright, symmetrical, and preceding every QRS except in missed beat
PRi	0.12–0.20 seconds
QRS	0.06–0.10 seconds

Causes

There are a number of potential causes of sinus block, which include MI; medications, such as digoxin; myocarditis; heart failure; carotid sinus sensitivity; and increased vagal tone. Sinus arrest is caused by similar factors but may also be caused by hyperkalemia, beta blockers, or calcium channel blockers.

Treatment

There is typically *no treatment required* for sinus block or sinus arrest unless there is hemodynamic compromise (e.g., significant hypotension).

Tips for Interpretation

Sinus arrest and sinus block appear as a missed beat or pause in the rhythm. This is how to tell them apart: Sinus block drops the beat and resets the rhythm right on time, whereas sinus arrest drops a beat but does not reset to the underlying rhythm at exactly two R–R intervals as sinus block does. In the case of a sinus block, the impulse arises normally in the sinoatrial (SA) node but is not transmitted. With a sinus arrest, the impulse fails to arise in the SA node and, therefore, there is also no transmission of the impulse.

Wandering Atrial Pacemaker

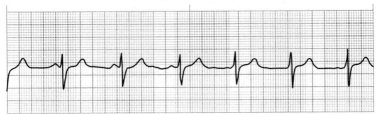

Figure 2.6 ■ Example of wandering atrial pacemaker.

Unique Characteristics

Rhythm	Regular or slightly irregular
Rate	60–100 beats/minute
P waves	**Vary in shape and size, one for every QRS**
PRi	0.12–0.20 seconds
QRS	0.06–0.10 seconds

Causes

This rhythm can be *seen in normal hearts* or during sleep. Occasionally, the wandering atrial pacemaker (WAP) rhythm can be caused by digoxin toxicity.

Treatment

No treatment required.

Tips for Interpretation

In the case of a wandering pacemaker, the pacemaker "wanders" between the SA node and the atria causing the impulses to be generated from a variety of locations in the atria. As the origin of where the impulse varies, this causes a **change in the shape and size of the P waves**. P waves in this rhythm are not the perfectly upright, rounded, and symmetrical P waves seen when all impulses arise directly from the SA node.

ATRIAL RHYTHMS

Atrial rhythms arise from an *irritable focus in the atria*. These rhythms can have significant effects for the patient hemodynamically and can result in the loss of atrial kick or a synchronized atrial contraction. The result of no atrial kick, for example, in the case of atrial flutter and atrial fibrillation, can result in a decrease in cardiac output of up to 30%. This drop in cardiac output can have serious effects on a patient's blood pressure, level of consciousness, and overall hemodynamic stability. In addition, when the atria are fluttering or fibrillating, mini clots can form in the atria and can cause serious consequences (e.g., stroke) if released. The first sign of trouble in the atria's electrical conduction system is when PACs begin to appear. These early ectopic beats superimposed on the underlying rhythm can transition very quickly into more dangerous atrial arrhythmias such as atrial flutter, atrial fibrillation, and SVT.

The primary cause of atrial arrhythmias includes factors such as overstretch or understretch (e.g., as with fluid overload or hypovolemia) of the atria and ischemia over the conduction system. Atrial arrhythmias must be identified and treated urgently to prevent further deterioration or sequelae (e.g., stroke, severe hypotension) in the patient.

Premature Atrial Contractions

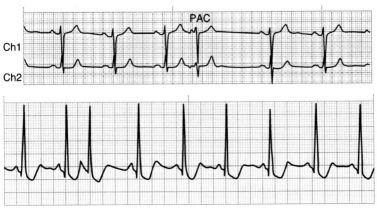

Figure 2.7 ▨ Examples of sinus rhythm with premature atrial contractions (PACs).

Unique Characteristics

Rhythm	Irregular because of the early beat (PAC) superimposed on the underlying rhythm
Rate	Usually 60–100 beats/minute in the underlying rhythm
P waves	P waves appear differently in the PAC versus the underlying sinus rhythm (as their origin is from the atria vs. the SA node).
PRi	0.12–0.20 seconds
QRS	0.06–0.10 seconds

Causes

Overall, atrial arrhythmias are caused by one of three underlying mechanisms: *altered automaticity, triggered activity,* or *reentry issues.* Altered automaticity can be caused by ischemia, drug toxicity, hypocalcemia, or hypoxia. Triggers can include such factors as ischemia, hypoxia, or low levels of magnesium. *Reentry issues that cause atrial arrhythmias can be initiated by hyperkalemia and some antiarrhythmics.* PACs are the first sign that there is irritability in the atria.

Treatment

Typically, there is *no treatment required* for PACs. The underlying cause should be treated and the frequency of PACs monitored because an increase in PACs indicates an increase in irritability of the atria and this could lead to a deterioration of the rhythm into a more dangerous atrial arrhythmia such as atrial fibrillation or SVT.

Tips for Interpretation

Watch for *early beats* with an upright P wave that looks slightly different than the underlying rhythm. Also, in some cases, the

P wave encroaches on the preceding T wave, causing the T wave on the preceding beat to look larger than the other T waves. If this occurs in the presence of an early beat with a normal QRS, we can assume the P is "buried" in the preceding T wave.

Atrial Flutter

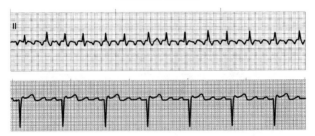

Figure 2.8 ■ Examples of atrial flutter.

Unique Characteristics

Rhythm	Regular or irregular
Rate	**Ventricular rate** (R–R) = 60–100 beats/minute (ventricular rate may be > 100 beats/minute, this is referred to as uncontrolled atrial) flutter. **Atrial rate** = 250–400 beats/minute
P waves	No "P" waves are present, instead **there are "F" waves or flutter waves**, which represent rapid atrial impulses.
PRi	There is no PRi (as there is no P wave) in this rhythm.
QRS	0.06–0.10 seconds

Causes

Causes of atrial flutter were discussed previously in overall causes of atrial arrhythmias. Specifically, conditions associated with atrial flutter include hypoxia, pulmonary embolism, pneumonia, chronic lung disease, coronary artery disease, MI, digoxin toxicity, myocarditis, or pericarditis. Patients who experience atrial flutter have a loss of atrial kick that can subsequently cause them to have palpitations, shortness of breath, fatigue, and chest discomfort caused by hypotension.

Treatment

Rate control is typically indicated as the priority treatment if the patient is stable. Rate control is typically achieved through use of beta blockers and calcium channel blockers such as diltiazem. Amiodarone may also be used, especially in the patient with heart failure. If the patient is *unstable* (particularly with accompanying high ventricular rates), *cardioversion* is recommended as the first-line treatment to halt the rhythm. Instability can manifest itself as severe hypotension, heart failure, or signs of shock. A discussion of cardioversion is found in Table 2.1. In addition, if the patient has been experiencing atrial flutter for more than 48 hours, the risk of emboli must be considered. Anticoagulants are recommended prior to cardioversion unless the patient is unstable and immediate electrical intervention is required (cardioversion).

Tips for Interpretation

In atrial flutter, there are no P waves; therefore, there is no PRi. Instead, there are flutter waves that are continuous and carry on right through the QRS. One of the key features of atrial flutter is the *"sawtooth" pattern of the flutter waves* making it a very distinctive looking rhythm. In order to calculate the ratio of flutter waves (e.g., atrial flutter with a 4:1 conduction), you must first calculate the ventricular rate and then calculate the atrial rate. If the R–R is irregular, this is referred to as a varying conduction. When the R–R is regular, the ventricular rate is divided into the atrial rate to calculate the conduction ratio. For example, if the ventricular (R–R) rate is 75 and the atrial rate is 300 (beginning of one flutter wave to beginning of the next) the conduction ratio is 4:1. *Please note:* You do not calculate the *conduction ratio* by counting the number of F (flutter) waves between R waves because flutter waves are continuous.

Atrial Fibrillation

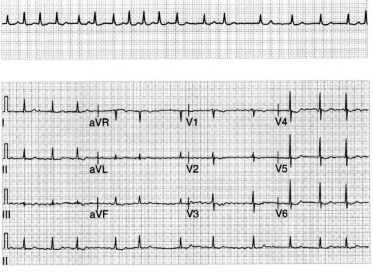

Figure 2.9 ■ Examples of atrial fibrillation.

Unique Characteristics

Rhythm	Irregular
Rate	**Ventricular rate:** 60–100 beats/minute (ventricular rate may be > 100 beats/minute, this is referred to as uncontrolled atrial fibrillation) **Atrial rate:** 400–600 beats/minute (This cannot be measured on the rhythm strip because the waveform is so chaotic.)
P waves	There are no P waves, instead there are **fibrillatory waves or "f" waves.**
PRi	There is no PRi since there is no P wave.
QRS	0.06–0.10 seconds

Causes

Atrial fibrillation is the most common type of arrhythmia. Causes of atrial fibrillation are similar to those of atrial flutter and produce similar signs and symptoms. Additional causes or triggers of atrial fibrillation can include excessive caffeine ingestion, idiopathic (no clear cause), increased age, stress, hypokalemia, infection, and hyperthyroidism.

Treatment

The treatment of atrial fibrillation is *similar to the treatment for atrial flutter* (see "Atrial Flutter" section). Ablation may be required for persistent, recurring atrial fibrillation. Ablation refers to a procedure that eliminates tissue through an energy source, such as a laser or cryothermy, with the goal of stopping the cause of the arrhythmia.

Tips for Interpretation

In atrial fibrillation, it is important to remember that the ventricular rhythm (R–R) is *always* irregular. Also, when naming the rhythm remember there is no such rhythm as atrial "fib/flutter." The patient may have runs of atrial flutter and then atrial fibrillation but they do not occur at the same time; therefore, each needs to be identified separately on the strip during interpretation.

Atrial Tachycardia (aka SVT or PSVT)

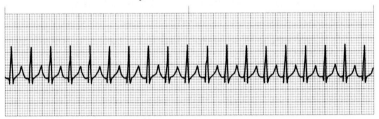

Figure 2.10 ■ Supraventricular tachycardia (SVT).

Unique Characteristics

Rhythm	Regular
Rate	150–250 beats/minute (usually closer to 200 and over)
P waves	Can be difficult to see when the rate is this fast
PRi	If you can see them, 0.12–0.20 seconds
QRS	0.06–0.10 seconds

Causes

Most SVTs are caused by reentry mechanisms which refer to the fact that the rhythm takes an abnormal repetitive circuit of cardiac tissue. Triggers can include *stimulants* (e.g., caffeine, albuterol), *infection, electrolyte imbalance*, or *MI*.

Treatment

Treatment for SVT includes consideration of *vagal maneuvers* (e.g., carotid sinus massage or having the patient bear down) and the administration of adenosine. *Adenosine* is initially given in a rapid 6-mg IV injection quickly followed by a 12-mg dose if the first was not successful. This medication creates almost a chemical type of "cardioversion" and has a very short half-life of only 10 to 15 seconds therefore the need for rapid administration. Upon administration of adenosine, it is advisable to inform the patient that they may initially feel uncomfortable and anxious but that this only lasts for a short period. Reassure the patient that the rhythm is being monitored closely and the reason for giving this medication. Should adenosine and vagal maneuvers fail to convert the rhythm, *calcium channel blockers* or *beta blockers* may be considered. If the patient is *unstable, immediate cardioversion* is indicated.

Tips for Interpretation

SVT *typically starts suddenly*, is preceded by a PAC, and the patient is often symptomatic (e.g., light headed, feeling "palpitations," flushed, or hypotensive). SVT is a broad term that can encompass paroxysmal atrial tachycardia or paroxysmal junctional tachycardia and refers to the fact that the "runaway" accessory path impulses are "supra," "ventricular," or originating above the ventricles.

Table 2.1 ▨ *Differentiating Cardioversion and Defibrillation*

	Cardioversion	Defibrillation
Definition	The delivery of a *synchronized* shock.	The delivery of an *asynchronized* shock.

(continued)

Table 2.1 ▪ *Differentiating Cardioversion and Defibrillation (continued)*

	Cardioversion	Defibrillation
Voltage	Initial shock usually begins low, 50–100 joules but may proceed (in increments) to the maximum voltage.	Initial shock is at maximum voltage (i.e., 360 joules in a monophasic unit, 120–200 joules in a biphasic unit).
Indications	Unstable SVT, atrial fibrillation, atrial flutter, ventricular tachycardia with a pulse. (consider sedation)	Ventricular fibrillation Pulseless ventricular tachycardia

EXERCISES

Case Study

You are working in the emergency department when Mr. T. (John), a 21-year-old male, is admitted at 7:00 a.m. John is a newly graduated RN and has been up "all night" and is "very stressed" after studying for the advanced cardiovascular life support course he must take in order to work in the intensive care unit. He states that he drank one pot of dark-roast coffee and had one energy drink at approximately 5:00 a.m. He started to feel unwell and says his chest feels like "palpitations" and he is a little light-headed. You attach the cardiac monitor and see the following rhythm. His vital signs are:

B/P (blood pressure) = 106/66

O_2 saturation = 95% on room air

Respiratory rate = 22

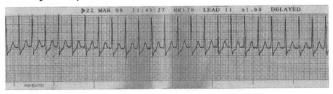

(continued)

(continued)

HR (heart rate) = 180
Temp = 37.1°C

1. Would you consider John to be stable or unstable at this point?
2. What rhythm is he in?
3. What is the priority treatment for this rhythm according to the current AHA guidelines?

Approximately 15 minutes after the initial treatment, John remains in the same rhythm and upon reassessment of his vital signs, his B/P is now 80/56 and he is losing consciousness.

4. What is the priority treatment for John at this point?

After this treatment is administered, John reverts to a rhythm that is regular, 80 beats/minute; PRi of 0.12 seconds; and QRS of 0.08 seconds.

5. What rhythm is John in now?
6. What are the likely causes of John's initial rhythm (on admission)?

Test Yourself!

---

1. What is the most common type of arrhythmia (and also one of the hardest to treat)?
   a. Sinus tachycardia
   b. Wandering atrial pacemaker
   c. Sinus block
   d. Atrial fibrillation
2. The drug of choice in a symptomatic bradycardia is:
   a. Adenosine
   b. Amiodarone

(continued)

(continued)

c. Atropine
d. Beta blocker
3. Treatment of sinus tachycardia includes:
a. Beta blockers
b. Pacing
c. Treating the cause
d. Cardioversion
4. Sinus arrhythmia is a benign rhythm and no treatment is required.
a. True
b. False
5. The definitive characteristic in WAP is:
a. An irregular rhythm
b. The P waves
c. The rate
d. The QRS duration

Practice Strips

Systematically interpret each rhythm.

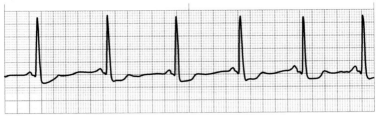

2.1

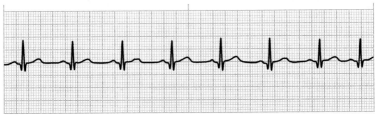

2.2

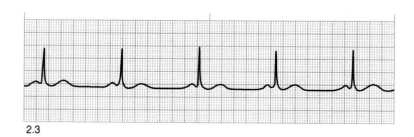

2.3

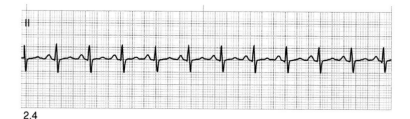

2.4

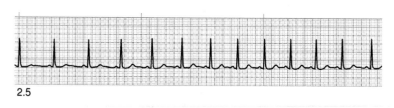

2.5

(See answers for Chapter 2 in the "Answers" chapter.)

RESOURCES

Aehlert, B. (2013). *ECGs made easy* (5th ed.). St. Louis, MO: Mosby.

American Heart Association. (2015). 2015 American Heart Association guidelines for cardiopulomonary resuscitation and emergency cardiac care. *Circulation, 132*(18, Suppl. 2), s313–s573. doi:10.1161/cir.00000000000261

Goldsworthy, S. (2012). *Coronary care 1 and 2 manual.* Oshawa, ON: Durham College Continuing Education.

Walraven, G. (2011). *Basic arrhythmias* (7th ed.). Toronto, ON: Pearson.

Arrhythmias: Junctional and Ventricular

JUNCTIONAL RHYTHMS

In this chapter, junctional and ventricular arrhythmias are discussed. Specifically, the following junctional rhythms are presented: premature junctional contractions (PJCs), junctional rhythm, accelerated junctional rhythm, and paroxysmal junctional tachycardia (PJT). The ventricular rhythms discussed are premature ventricular contractions (PVCs), ventricular tachycardia (VT), ventricular fibrillation (VF), idioventricular rhythm, accelerated idioventricular rhythm (AIVR), and agonal rhythm. The unique characteristics of each are provided along with causes, treatment, tips for interpretation, and practice examples. Finally, a case study and "test yourself" questions are provided to help you differentiate among rhythms quickly and accurately.

Junctional rhythms are a group of arrhythmias that are mostly benign (in other words they are typically not lethal!) and often transient. The primary pacemaker for these rhythms is the atrioventricular (AV) node, whereas the normal pacemaker for the heart is the sinoatrial (SA) node. A common characteristic of all junctional rhythms is the presence of inverted (or absent) P waves. This irregularity occurs because of retrograde conduction, in other words, the impulse has to go backward to be able to depolarize the atria because the impulse is arising in the AV node rather than the SA node–the normal pacemaker of the heart. Because the conduction is retrograde, from the AV node to the atria, depolarization can occur prior to the ventricles being depolarized, which would result in three possible configurations: (a) an inverted P wave prior to the QRS; (b) a P wave that is not seen because the atria are depolarized close to the same time the ventricles are depolarized; and (c) an inverted P wave seen after the QRS, indicating that the impulse traveled to the ventricles first and then subsequently depolarized the atria.

The primary causes of junctional rhythms are drug toxicity (e.g., digoxin) or ischemia. Once the toxicity is resolved or the area reperfuses, typically the junctional rhythm converts to a sinus rhythm. This grouping of rhythms is identified by similar characteristics (inverted or absent P's in the presence of a normal duration QRS) and the rhythms are named or defined according to their rates. Junctional rhythm is the slowest; its impulses are generated at the expected rate at which the AV node fires: 40 to 60 impulses per minute. Accelerated junctional rhythm is faster, and is followed by PJT, which has the fastest rate of all the junctional rhythms.

PJCs are early ectopic beats that arise from the AV node. As with premature atrial contractions (PACs), these beats indicate that there is an issue with the AV node and may lead to other junctional rhythms if the problem or underlying cause continues. Specifics of each of the junctional rhythms are discussed in the following text along with examples and practice strips.

Helpful Tips

Unique characteristics of each rhythm that help differentiate it from others appear in **bold face**.

Premature Junctional Contractions

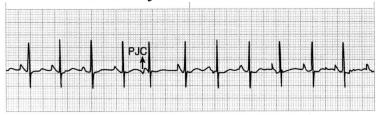

Figure 3.1 ■ Premature junctional contraction.

Unique Characteristics

Rhythm	Irregular as a result of early beat (PJC)
Rate	Underlying rhythm is typically 60–100 beats/minute
P waves	**Inverted or absent**; may be seen before, during, or after the QRS
PRi (PR interval)	Shortened; not relevant because conduction is altered and retrograde
QRS	0.06–0.10 seconds

Causes

Causes of PJCs can include (but are not limited to) heart failure, fatigue, electrolyte imbalance, digoxin toxicity, rheumatic heart disease, and *stimulants* such as caffeine, cocaine, and tobacco.

Treatment

Typically, there is *no treatment required* for PJCs. The underlying cause should be treated and the frequency of PJCs monitored as an increase in PJCs indicates an increase in irritability of the AV node/junctional tissue; this could lead to a deterioration of the rhythm into a more significant arrhythmia such as junctional rhythm.

Tips for Interpretation

PJCs are *early beats* that can be easily confused with PACs. Here are some tips to keep them straight: PJCs have *inverted or absent P waves*. PJCs do not cause an increase in the amplitude of the preceding T wave as PACs can because PJCs do not have an upright P wave that can encroach on the T.

Junctional Rhythm

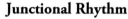

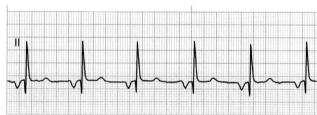

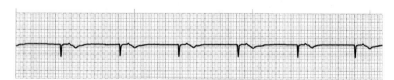

Figure 3.2 ■ Two examples of junctional rhythm.

Unique Characteristics

Rhythm	Regular
Rate	**40–60 beats/minute**
P waves	**Inverted (or absent)**; may be seen before, during, or after the QRS
PRi	Not relevant since there is retrograde conduction
QRS	0.06–0.10 seconds

Causes

Causes of junctional rhythm are similar to those that cause PJCs but can also include SA node disease; medications, such as beta blockers and calcium channel blockers; and increased parasympathetic tone.

Treatment

Treatment for this rhythm includes *treating the cause* because the patient is typically asymptomatic in this rhythm.

Tips for Interpretation

The key to identifying junctional rhythms is noting the presence of an *inverted P wave*, which can occur before or after the QRS. If the *P* wave is occurring during the QRS, it will not be seen.

Accelerated Junctional Rhythm

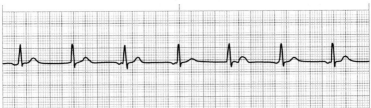

Figure 3.3 ■ Accelerated junctional rhythm.

Unique Characteristics

Rhythm	Regular
Rate	**60–100 beats/minute**
P waves	**Inverted or not seen**; may be seen before, during, or after the QRS
PRi	Not relevant because there is retrograde conduction
QRS	0.06–0.10 seconds

Causes

The most common culprits inciting this rhythm include digoxin toxicity and cardiac ischemia. Other causes can include chronic obstructive pulmonary disease (COPD) and hypokalemia.

Treatment

Treatment for this rhythm includes *treating the cause* (e.g., holding digoxin if this is the suspected cause) because the patient is typically asymptomatic in this rhythm.

Tips for Interpretation

Once again, key characteristics to watch for in junctional rhythms *are inverted P waves.* In addition, *note the rate* as this will define whether it is a junctional rhythm (slower = 40–60 beats/minute) or an accelerated junctional rhythm (faster = 60–100 beats/ minute). In some clinical areas, a separate category of junctional rhythms is referred to and this is called *junctional tachycardia*, which has the same characteristics as accelerated junctional rhythm and junctional rhythm but has a faster rate (100–140 beats/minute). For the purposes of this text, junctional tachycardia is not included as a common term.

Junctional Tachycardia

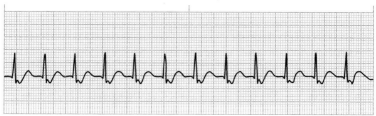

Figure 3.4 ▨ Junctional tachycardia.

Unique Characteristics

Rhythm	Regular
Rate	101–180 beats/minute
P waves	Inverted or not seen; may be seen before, during, or after the QRS
PRi	Not relevant as there is retrograde conduction
QRS	0.06–0.10 seconds

Causes

This rhythm is rarely seen and is thought to occur as a result of increased automaticity. It may be seen in conditions such as heart failure, acute coronary syndrome (ACS), and with digoxin toxicity.

Treatment

Vagal maneuvers and *adenosine* may be attempted initially if the patient is stable. Should the patient become *unstable*, immediate *cardioversion* is recommended. If the patient is a candidate, beta blockers or calcium channel blockers may be utilized if initial treatment is ineffective.

Tips for Interpretation

There are two types of junctional tachycardia: nonparoxysmal and paroxysmal. The first characteristics to note about the paroxysmal type of junctional tachycardia rhythm are that it typically *starts very suddenly* and can be very difficult to differentiate from paroxysmal atrial tachycardia because the P waves become "buried" in the rhythm. If the differentiation cannot be made or the PJC that initiated the rhythm cannot be identified, the rhythm is then often referred to as *supra VT*.

VENTRICULAR RHYTHMS

Ventricular arrhythmias are among the easiest to identify, which is a good thing as they are often lethal if not treated quickly. What makes them easier to spot is the wide, bizarre QRS complex (> 0.12 seconds), which is a hallmark sign of ventricular arrhythmias. In addition to the wide QRS complex present with each of these rhythms, the P wave is absent.

There are essentially two "groupings" of ventricular rhythms. The first group of ventricular arrhythmias is caused by irritability within the ventricle. Many factors can cause this irritability such as hypoxemia, acid–base imbalance, hypothermia, and electrolyte imbalance (abnormally high or low levels of potassium, calcium, and magnesium). Initially, when the ventricle becomes irritated, PVCs can result. PVCs are a sign that the ventricle is beginning to get irritated. If the cause continues, PVCs can quickly deteriorate into the lethal rhythms of VT and VF. Underlying causes need to be considered and treated quickly to prevent more dangerous rhythms from occurring. There are a number of different configurations that PVCs can have. For instance, PVCs may be uniform (all look the same); these beats are called unifocal PVCs, which are different than multifocal PVCs, as these vary in shape and are more dangerous because they indicate that there are multiple irritable foci within the ventricle. Three or more PVCs together are classified as VT and two PVCs together are referred to as "couplets." Another term that is frequently used with PVCs is bigeminy (PVCs are occurring every second beat) or trigeminy (PVCs occur every third beat). These terms are important when documenting the patient's rhythm or providing a hand-off report. VT is differentiated from VF by having a regular rhythm with wide QRS complexes, whereas VF has a chaotic, irregular rhythm with no QRS complexes present. Both rhythms require immediate life-saving treatment, which will be discussed in the following section.

The next grouping of ventricular rhythms, which includes idioventricular rhythm, AIVR, and aganol rhythm, are caused by failure of higher level pacemakers (i.e., SA node and AV node). Once these pacemakers have failed, the ventricle "takes over" as the default pacemaker for the heart. Because the ventricle is only capable of discharging impulses at a very slow rate (typically < 40 beats/minute), the rates of these rhythms are very slow. In addition, because atrial kick is lost, the cardiac output also tends to be quite low with these rhythms. Because these rhythms are not caused by irritability as in the case of VF or VT, the treatment is quite different. For instance, should ventricular antiarrhythmics be administered to these rhythms, they could cause complete loss of a pacemaker for the heart and asystole could potentially result. Therefore, ventricular antiarrhythmic medications, such as amiodarone, should *never* be administered for idioventricular or AIVRs.

Premature Ventricular Contractions

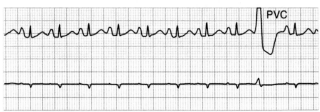

(continued)

(continued)

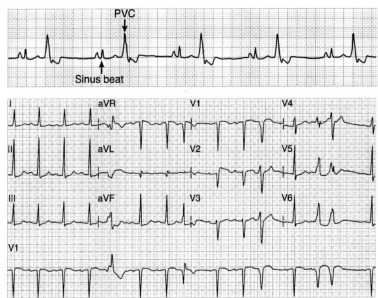

Figure 3.5 ■ Three examples of premature ventricular contractions (PVCs).

Unique Characteristics

Rhythm	Irregular as a result of the **early beat** (PVC)
Rate	Underlying rhythm rate can vary, usually 60–100 beats/minute.
P waves	None in PVC
PRi	None in PVC (since no P wave)
QRS	**Wide and bizarre** (> 0.12 seconds) in PVC

Causes

There are many causes of PVCs. Here are some of the more common ones:

■ Stimulants (e.g., caffeine)
■ Stress/anxiety

■ Electrolyte of acid–base imbalance
■ Cardiac ischemia
■ Hypoxia
■ Increased sympathetic tone
■ Medications such as tricyclic antidepressants, sympathomimetics (e.g., dopamine)

Treatment

Typically, there is *no treatment required* for PVCs. The underlying cause should be treated and the frequency of PVCs monitored because an increase in PVCs indicates an increase in irritability of the ventricle, which this could lead to a deterioration of the rhythm into a much more dangerous or lethal arrhythmia such as VF. It is important to note the configuration of the PVCs as some are more dangerous than others.

Tips for Interpretation

These early beats can be easily seen because of the wide and bizarre configuration of the QRS. Here is a reminder of the terminology used for PVCs:

> *Unifocal PVCs* = all PVCs in the rhythm look identical (least dangerous type since they come from one focus)
> *Multifocal PVCs* = PVCs that have different configurations (they look different); these are more dangerous than unifocal PVCs because the impulses are coming from different irritable foci
> *Couplets* = two PVCs that occur together
> *Bigeminy* = every other beat is a PVC
> *Trigeminy* = every third beat is a PVC

■ Remember, *three PVCs together* = a "run" of VT. When documenting be sure to add the number of beats present in a short burst of VT (e.g., the patient had a run of 16 beats of VT) or, if it is a prolonged run, this is referred to as a sustained run of VT.

VT: Monomorphic

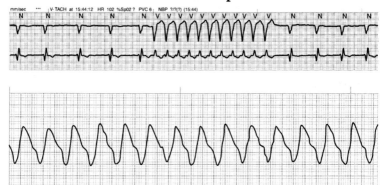

Figure 3.6 ■ Two examples of ventricular tachycardia.

Unique Characteristics

Rhythm	Regular
Rate	150–250 beats/minute
P waves	Absent
PRi	None
QRS	**Wide and bizarre**, > 0.12 seconds

Clinical Pearls	There is also another type of VT called *polymorphic VT* (or Torsades de pointes—"twisting of the points"). With this type of tachycardia, rhythm may be irregular or regular with an alteration in the amplitude and direction of the QRS. Polymorphic VT is typically resistant to the traditional treatment of VT and often results from low levels of magnesium. Treatment requires intravenous (IV) *administration of magnesium* at doses of 1 to 2 g.

Causes (Monomorphic VT)

Causes are similar to those listed under PVCs (see earlier) but can also include cocaine abuse and trauma such as myocardial contusion or cardiomyopathy.

Treatment

VT can be a lethal rhythm and needs to be treated immediately. It is important to quickly determine whether the patient has a pulse or not because VT can present with or without a pulse. In fact, a person could be awake and talking to you and be in VT.

Treatment of VT Without a Pulse

First things first (for in-hospital arrests): Approach the patient using American Heart Association (AHA, 2015) guidelines using circulation, airway, and breathing (CAB):

1. If the patient is not visibly breathing proceed to Step 2.
2. Immediately establish whether the patient has a pulse or not.
3. If not—call a code blue (cardiac arrest) to ensure the cardiac arrest team is on the way.
4. Begin compressions at a rate of 30:2 (compressions to ventilations).
5. Manage the airway using two responders: one to insert the oropharyngeal airway and create the seal with the resuscitation bag and the other to manually ventilate and ensure the resuscitation bag is connected to oxygen.
6. As soon as a defibrillator is available the patient should be defibrillated and high-quality cardiopulmonary resuscitation (CPR) continued.
7. A 1-mg IV of epinephrine is the first medication that will be given in the arrest if the rhythm is not converted after the second shock (defibrillation).

8. Subsequent medications include 300-mg IV of amiodarone and repetition of the epinephrine every 3 to 5 minutes. If the amiodarone is required again, the second dose is administered at 150-mg IV.

9. Potential causes of VT must be considered and the underlying cause treated to improve the likelihood of return of spontaneous circulation (ROSC).

Treatment of VT With a Pulse

In the event that the patient in VT has a pulse, cardioversion beginning at 100 J, and the administration of amiodarone beginning at 150-mg IV are the treatments of choice.

Tips for Interpretation

The key to differentiating VT from VF is that monomorphic VT has a *regular rhythm* with wide, bizarre QRS complexes, whereas VF has a chaotic baseline with no discernible QRS complexes.

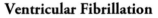

Ventricular Fibrillation

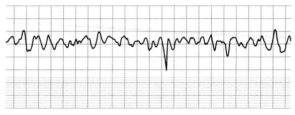

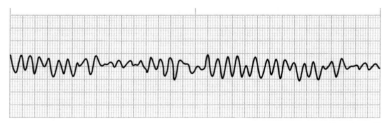

(continued)

(continued)

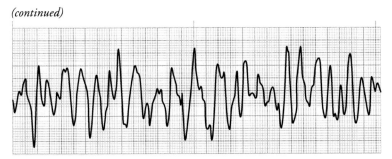

Figure 3.7 ■ Three examples of ventricular fibrillation.

Unique Characteristics

Rhythm	Chaotic, irregular
Rate	Cannot be counted (no discernible waves)
P waves	None
PRi	None
QRS	None discernible

Causes

See previously mentioned causes of VT.

Treatment

See VT with *no* pulse treatment; the treatment for VF is identical.

Tips for Interpretation

VF is likely the easiest rhythm to spot because it is *chaotic with no discernible QRS complexes*. Good thing, because this rhythm needs to be responded to with utmost speed! The longer the patient has been in ventricular rhythm, the finer this wave becomes (and also the more difficult to successfully treat). This rhythm typically starts out as coarse VF and proceeds into a waveform with reduced amplitude.

Clinical Pearls	*Potential Causes of Cardiac Arrest: 5 Hs and 5 Ts*	
	Hypovolemia	Tamponade
	Hypoxia	Tension pneumothorax
	Hypothermia	Thrombosis: lungs
	Hypokalemia/ hyperkalemia	Thrombosis: heart
	Hydrogen ion (acidosis)	Tablets/toxins: drug overdose
	Source: AHA (2015).	

Idioventricular Rhythm

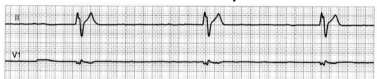

Figure 3.8 ▨ Idioventricular rhythm.

Unique Characteristics

Rhythm	Regular
Rate	**< 40 beats/minute**
P waves	None

(continued)

(continued)

PRi	None
QRS	**Wide and bizarre**

Causes

Failure of supraventricular pacemakers can cause this rhythm. Idioventricular rhythm can also be seen as a *reperfusion arrhythmia* after the administration of a thrombolytic medication. Occasionally, myocardial infarction (MI) and digoxin toxicity can cause this rhythm.

Treatment

This rhythm is usually transient and no treatment is typically required. It is critical to note that ventricular antiarrhythmic drugs, such as *lidocaine, are contraindicated* in this rhythm because, if administered, they could rapidly cause asystole.

Tips for Interpretation

As with all ventricular rhythms, idioventricular rhythm has *wide, bizarre QRS complexes* but its rate is *much slower* than the rhythms caused by ventricular irritability.

Accelerated Idioventricular Rhythm

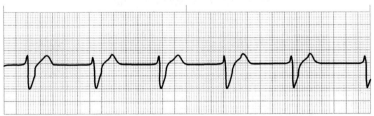

Figure 3.9 ■ Accelerated idioventricular rhythm.

Unique Characteristics

Rhythm	Regular
Rate	41–100 beats/minute
P waves	None
PRi	None
QRS	Wide and bizarre

Causes

▩ Same as idioventricular rhythm (see earlier)

Treatment

▩ Same as idioventricular rhythm (see earlier)

Tips for Interpretation

AIVR *looks almost identical to idioventricular rhythm*; the only difference is that the *rate is slightly faster*.

Aganol Rhythm (aka "Dying Heart" Rhythm)

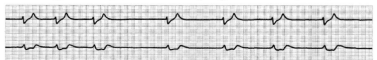

Figure 3.10 ▩ Aganol rhythm.

Unique Characteristics

Rhythm	**Irregular**
Rate	Often < 20 beats/minute

(continued)

(continued)

P waves	None
PRi	None
QRS	**Wide and bizarre**, often with decreasing amplitude

Causes

■ End-stage cardiac disease

Treatment

This rhythm is refractory to treatment and occurs at the end stage of cardiac disease; it usually represents the last bit of electrical activity in the heart and is associated with very little cardiac output.

Tips for Interpretation

As indicated, this rhythm often represents the last remaining electrical activity in the heart and is accompanied by very little cardiac output. As a result, this rhythm looks almost like it is "fading out"; it becomes *slower, often wider, and has decreased amplitude.*

EXERCISES

Case Study

Mrs. L. is a 62-year-old patient on a medicine telemetry floor. She was admitted with an anterior MI. She has a previous history of a lateral MI 1 year ago for which she received two stents. She is due to be discharged today. You proceed into her room to complete a final assessment. As you approach her, she does not respond to her name and is visibly not breathing.

(continued)

(continued)

1. What is your immediate priority intervention?

   A code blue is called and the cardiac arrest team arrives and connects her to the monitor. CPR is in progress. She is in the following rhythm:

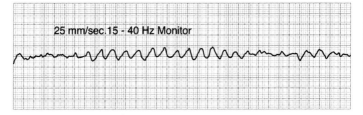

2. What rhythm is this?
3. What is the definitive immediate treatment required for this rhythm?

   Mrs. L. continues in this rhythm.
4. What is the first drug administered for this rhythm and at what time point is it given?
5. Should Mrs. L. have ROSC? What would be your immediate priority interventions?

Test Yourself!

1. Defibrillation is used to treat which two rhythms only?
2. Match the following (cardioversion [C] or defibrillation [D])
   a. Voltage starts at maximum energy
   b. Asynchronized shock
   c. Used to treat unstable supraventricular tachycardia
   d. Used to treat pulseless VT

(continued)

(continued)

> **3.** PVCs are caused by an irritable focus in the ventricles. Name the following types:
> a. All look the same
> b. They have different configurations
> c. Two together
> d. Every other beat is a PVC
> **4.** Lidocaine must *never* be given to someone in an idioventricular rhythm.
> a. True
> b. False
> **5.** This is the first drug given in a VF arrest (after the second defibrillation).

Practice Strips

Systematically interpret each rhythm.

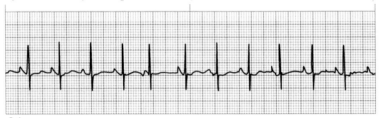

3.1

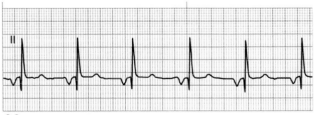

3.2

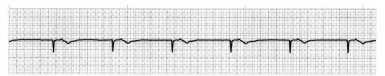

3.3

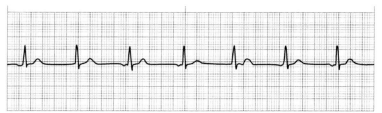

3.4

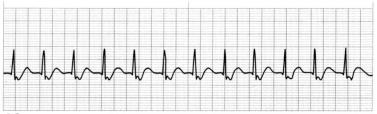

3.5

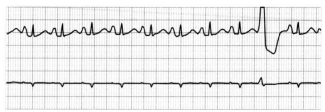

3.6

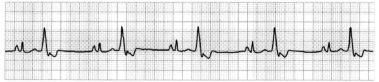

3.7

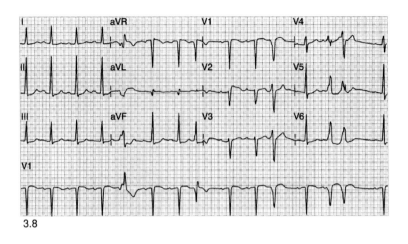

3.8

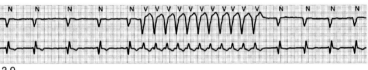

3.9

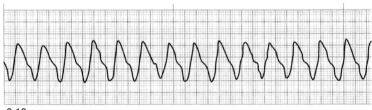

3.10

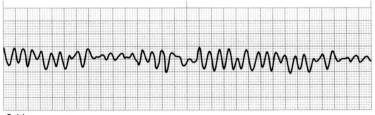

3.11

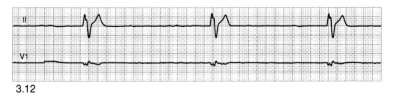

3.12

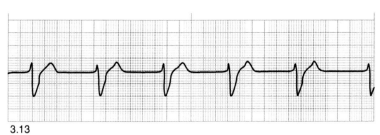

3.13

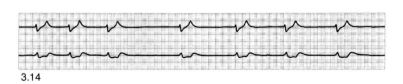

3.14

(See answers for Chapter 3 in the "Answers" chapter.)

RESOURCES

Aehlert, B. (2013). *ECGs made easy* (5th ed.). St. Louis, MO: Mosby.

American Heart Association. (2015). 2015 American Heart Association guidelines for cardiopulmonary resuscitation and emergency cardiac care. *Circulation*, *132*(18 Suppl. 2), s313–s573. doi:10.1161/cir.00000000000261

Goldsworthy, S. (2012). *Coronary care 1 and 2 manual*. Oshawa, ON: Durham College Continuing Education.

Walraven, G. (2011). *Basic arrhythmias* (7th ed.). Toronto, ON: Pearson.

4

Arrhythmias: Atrioventricular Blocks

ATRIOVENTRICULAR BLOCKS

There are four atrioventricular (AV) blocks that will be discussed in this section: first-degree AV block, second-degree Type I, second-degree Type II, and third-degree or complete heart block. Of the four AV blocks, two are typically benign (first-degree and second-degree Type I) and do not usually cause hemodynamic consequences, whereas the other two (second-degree Type II and third-degree AV block) can be lethal and typically require emergency treatment.

There is a simple analogy that you can use when trying to sort out which AV block is which. I relate this to a doorman in an apartment building and callers coming to the door, each ringing the doorbell. Imagine that you have a doorman and several people who ring the bell at the apartment building. In the first instance, the person rings the doorbell and the door-man takes a little longer to answer the door. Each time some-one rings, the doorman is delayed; he always takes the same amount of time to answer the door. This is like first-degree AV block; the caller (the sinoatrial [SA] node in the case of the heart) rings the doorbell but the doorman (the AV node) is delayed in answering (therefore, the PRi [PR interval] is prolonged > 0.20 seconds and, because the delay is always the same, the prolonged interval is constant).

In the case of a second-degree Type I AV block, the doorman takes longer to answer the door each time (PRi gradually gets longer) until he decides to not answer the door (a beat is dropped) and then the cycle continues.

Using our analogy in the case of a second-degree Type II heart block, imagine the caller ringing the doorbell and the doorman taking the same amount of time to answer the door each time but once in a while (randomly) he decides not to answer the door at all (a randomly dropped beat).

Last, in a third-degree AV block, the callers keep ringing the doorbell but our doorman decides not to answer the door at all but rather to continue on with his own activities on the other side of the door. In other words, the SA node continues to fire at its usual rate (60–100 beats/minute) and the ventricles carry on with their own rhythm and rate, each working independently.

The key characteristics, causes, treatment, and tips for interpretation are described to help you differentiate among the four AV blocks.

> ### Helpful Tips
>
> Unique characteristics of each rhythm that help differentiate it from others appear in **bold face**.

First-Degree AV Block

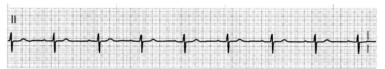

(continued)

(continued)

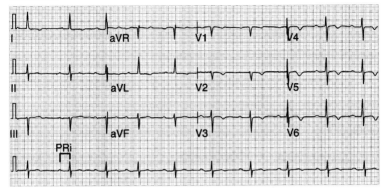

Figure 4.1 ■ Two examples of first-degree heart block.

Unique Characteristics

Rhythm	Regular
Rate	60–100 beats/minute
P waves	Upright, symmetrical, one for every QRS
PRi	**Prolonged > 0.20 seconds**
QRS	0.06–0.10 seconds

Causes

First-degree heart block can be a normal finding in some people but other causes include ischemia to the AV node area, rheumatic heart disease, myocardial infarction (MI), increased vagal tone, or increased potassium.

Treatment

Treatment is not required for first-degree heart block as it is typically asymptomatic. It is important, however, to continue to monitor for an increasing block, which can occur with prolonged ischemia at the AV node/junctional tissue area.

Tips for Interpretation

First-degree heart block looks identical to normal sinus rhythm with one key difference; the *PRi is prolonged (> 0.20 seconds) and constant.*

Second-Degree AV Block Type I (aka Wenkebach)

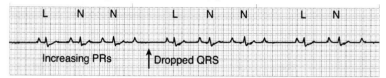

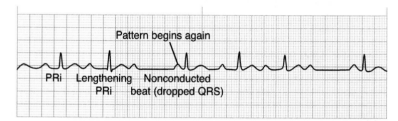

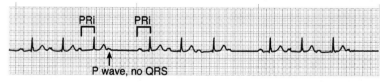

Figure 4.2 ▓ Three examples of second-degree Type I AV block (Wenkebach).

Unique Characteristics

Rhythm	Irregular
Rate	Ventricular rate usually 60–100 beats/minute
P waves	Present, upright, symmetrical, one for every QRS (except dropped beat)
PRi	**Gradually lengthens** until a beat is dropped
QRS	0.06–0.10 seconds

Causes

Ischemia or increased parasympathetic tone can cause second-degree Type I (Wenkebach) rhythm.

Treatment

This rhythm is benign and typically transient; therefore, no treatment is required. Patients are not typically symptomatic with this rhythm.

Tips for Interpretation

The main way to distinguish second-degree heart block Type I from all of the other AV blocks is that the *PRi progressively lengthens* until a beat is dropped. The rhythm resets and the process begins again.

Second-Degree AV Block Type II (aka Mobitz II)

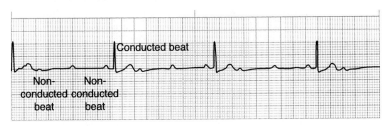

Figure 4.3 ■ Second-degree Type I AV heart block.

Unique Characteristics

Rhythm	Irregular R–R (or regular if 2:1 block present)
Rate	Ventricular rate can vary but is often < 60 beats/minute Atrial rate typically 60–100 beats/minute

(continued)

(continued)

P waves	More Ps than QRS waves
PRi	0.12–0.20, constant
QRS	Can be widened or within normal parameters (0.06–0.10 seconds)

Causes

Disease of the left coronary artery (LCA) or an anterior MI can cause this rhythm.

Treatment

Treatment of this rhythm involves *transcutaneous pacing* or a *vasopressor infusion* (e.g., dopamine or epinephrine) to increase the rate and improve the cardiac output. If the conduction system does not adequately perfuse, a permanent pacemaker may need to be inserted. See Chapter 5 for a discussion of pacemakers and paced rhythms. Atropine administration is not effective in this rhythm.

Tips for Interpretation

Differentiating second-degree Type II from third-degree heart block can be tricky for new learners. Both rhythms have more P waves than QRS complexes and in both cases QRS complexes can be of normal duration or widened (> 0.12 seconds). Here are the key differences to watch for between the two rhythms: In second-degree heart block wherever there is a *P that coincides with a QRS*, the PRi is constant (it may or may not be prolonged but it is *always constant*, which means the duration is the same in all beats), whereas in third-degree or complete heart block, there is never a relationship between the P waves and the QRS complexes. In other words, the PRi is not related to the QRS (i.e., the atria and ventricle are functioning independently).

Complete Heart Block (Third-Degree Block)

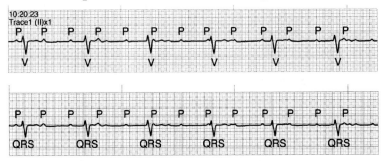

Figure 4.4 ■ Third-degree AV block (complete heart block).

Unique Characteristics

Rhythm	R–R regular P–P regular but P waves are not related to QRS (dissociated)
Rate	Ventricular rate typically < 60 beats/minute but can be faster Atrial rate 60–100 beats/minute
P waves	More Ps that QRS waves
PRi	Varied, no relationship to QRS
QRS	Widened or within normal limits (0.06–0.10 seconds)

Causes

This rhythm is often associated with an *inferior MI*, ischemia, or an anterior MI.

Treatment

Treatment of this rhythm involves *transcutaneous pacing* or a *vasopressor infusion* (e.g., dopamine or epinephrine) to increase the rate and improve the cardiac output. If the conduction system does not adequately perfuse, a permanent pacemaker may need to be inserted. See Chapter 5 for a discussion of pacemakers and paced rhythms. Atropine administration is not effective in this rhythm.

Tips for Interpretation

The key characteristic in third-degree heart block is that the *P–P is regular and the R–R is regular but the P wave and QRS are not related.* In practice, we say "the Ps march right through" meaning that the SA node continues to generate P waves at a rate of 60 to 100 regardless of what the ventricles are doing, and the ventricles carry on with their own rhythm and rate. There is no communication between the two because the AV node is "completely blocked" and not functional. It is important to note that in third-degree heart block, the QRS may be normal or widened. Do not be "put off the trail" because the QRS is of normal duration.

EXERCISES

Case Study

You are working in the emergency department when Mr. J., a 72-year-old male, is admitted. He states that he feels light-headed, very "sweaty" and more "tired" than usual. He is accompanied by his wife, who tells you that he has been treated on and off for "chest pain." He has taken all his medications this morning, which include a beta blocker, ASA (acetylsalicylic acid), and an ACE (angiotensin-converting enzyme) inhibitor. As you are speaking to him he becomes less alert and is not as responsive to questions.

(continued)

(continued)

On assessment his vital signs are:

Heart rate (HR) = 42
Blood pressure (B/P) = 82/42
Respiratory rate = 20
O₂ saturation = 93% on room air
Temperature = 36.6°C

He is in the following rhythm:

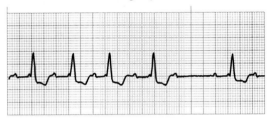

1. What rhythm is Mr. J. in?
2. Is he stable or unstable at this point?
3. What is the required priority treatment? What other options are recommended?
4. Would atropine be effective in this rhythm?
5. What are potential causes of this rhythm?

Test Yourself!

1. The treatment for third-degree heart block includes:
   a. Transcutaneous pacemaker or dopamine infusion
   b. Beta blockers and an epinephrine infusion
   c. Oxygen and cardioversion
   d. No treatment is required, continue to monitor
2. This is the key characteristic in second-degree Type I AV block.

(continued)

(continued)

3. Atropine is typically ineffective in second-degree Type II AV block and third-degree block.
   a. True
   b. False
4. These are the two AV blocks that *do not* require urgent treatment.
5. How do you differentiate between a third-degree heart block and second-degree, Type II AV block?

Practice Strips

Systematically interpret each rhythm.

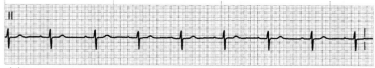

4.1

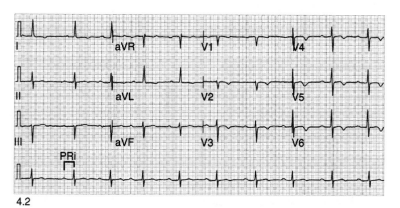

4.2

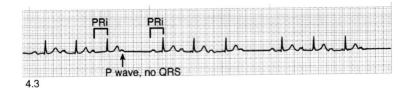

4.3

(See answers for Chapter 4 in the "Answers" chapter.)

RESOURCES

Aehlert, B. (2011). *ECGs made easy* (4th ed.). St. Louis, MO: Mosby.

American Heart Association. (2015). 2015 American Heart Association guidelines for cardiopulomonary resuscitation and emergency cardiac care. *Circulation, 132*(18, Suppl. 2), s313–s573. doi:10.1161/cir.00000000000261

Diehl, T. (Ed.). (2011). *ECG interpretation made incredibly easy!* Philadelphia, PA: Wolters Kluwer Lippincott Williams & Wilkins.

Goldsworthy, S. (2012). *Coronary care 1 and 2 manual.* Oshawa, ON: Durham College Continuing Education.

Walraven, G. (2011). *Basic arrhythmias* (7th ed.). Toronto, ON: Pearson.

5

Arrhythmias: Asystole, Pulseless Electrical Activity, and Paced Rhythms

In this chapter, asystole, pulseless electrical activity (PEA), and paced rhythms are discussed. Paced rhythms are further described in terms of oversensing, undersensing, and failure to pace. The unique characteristics of each of these arrhythmias along with causes, treatment, tips for interpretation, and practice examples are provided. Finally, a case study and "test yourself" questions are offered to help you quickly and accurately differentiate among rhythms.

Asystole and PEA are both life-threatening rhythms that are associated with the absence of a pulse and require emergency treatment. The primary causes of and treatment for asystole and PEA are discussed in the following section.

Paced rhythms can also be associated with significant hemodynamic instability and loss of cardiac output if the rate is inadequate, pacemaker malfunction occurs, the heart can't be paced effectively because of ischemia or infarct or because specific medications impact the contractile function of the heart.

Helpful Tips

Unique characteristics of each rhythm that help differentiate it from others appear in **bold face**.

PULSELESS RHYTHMS

Asystole

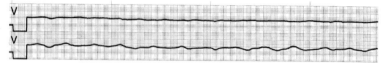

Figure 5.1 ■ Asystole.

Unique Characteristics

Rhythm	Absent
Rate	Absent
P waves	Absent
PRi (PR interval)	Absent
QRS	Absent ("flat line")

Causes

Asystole is most commonly seen following ventricular fibrillation or asystole. Resuscitation is far more unlikely than in other pulseless rhythms.

Treatment

Immediate treatment is indicated for this rhythm because it is life threatening and must be converted as quickly as possible. Once pulselessness is established, cardiopulmonary resuscitation (CPR) should be established immediately. To maintain the effectiveness of compressions, providers should be switched at 2-minute intervals and a pulse check performed if an organized rhythm emerges. The rhythm should be assessed every 2 minutes. One milligram of epinephrine should be administered intravenously/intraosseously (IV/IO) every 3 to 5 minutes while in asystole.

Tips for Interpretation

Luckily, asystole is very easy to recognize because of the "flat line" nature of the rhythm as it has no P waves or QRS complexes. If there is a small undulation in the presenting rhythm and it is difficult to distinguish between asystole and fine ventricular fibrillation, always treat as ventricular fibrillation until proven otherwise.

Pulseless Electrical Activity

Unique Characteristics

Rhythm	Varies
Rate	Varies
P waves	Varies
PRi	Varies
QRS	0.06–0.10 seconds (usually)

Causes

Causes of PEA are similar to the causes of asystole but can also include a variety of clinical situations such as hypovolemia or hypoxia (see Table 5.1 for further details).

Treatment

Immediate treatment is indicated for this rhythm because it is life threatening and must be converted as quickly as possible. Treatment for PEA is similar to treatment for asystole. In addition, reversible causes should be considered. Common causes of PEA include hypoxia, hypovolemia, pulmonary embolism, tension pneumothorax, acidosis, hypo-/hyperkalemia, hypothermia, toxins, cardiac thrombosis, and pulmonary thrombosis.

Should resuscitation be successful and there is return of spontaneous circulation (ROSC), care should be focused on treating the hypotension, hypoxemia, and the cause of the arrhythmia. Therapeutic hypothermia should be considered when the patient is in a comatose state after ROSC.

Tips for Interpretation

The key to identifying PEA rhythms is noting the presence or absence of a pulse. If a pulse is present, then PEA can be ruled out.

Table 5.1 ▧ *Causes of Pulseless Electrical Activity/Asystole*

Hypovolemia	Tension pneumothorax
Hypoxemia	Cardiac tamponade
Acidosis	Toxins
Hypo-/hyperkalemia	Pulmonary thrombosis
Hypothermia	Cardiac thrombosis

PACEMAKER RHYTHMS

Pacemakers deliver an electrical impulse to the heart with the goal of causing depolarization. Common indications for pacemakers include symptomatic bradycardias (i.e., third-degree atrioventricular [AV] block, second-degree Type II AV block) and symptomatic sinus bradycardia. Typical components of a pacemaker include a pulse generator (power source) and a pacing lead that is in contact with the endocardium. Although there are several different types of pacemakers that are permanent or temporary, this section focuses on temporary pacemakers (temporary transvenous or transcutaneous pacemakers) in the acute clinical situation.

Transcutaneous Pacemakers

Transcutaneous pacemakers are used in short-term, emergency situations. They consist of a power source and pacemaker pads that are attached to the chest in either the anterior/posterior ("heart sandwich") position or on the anterior chest with one pad placed just below the right clavicle and to the right of the sternum and the second pad placed to the left of the sternum at the midclavicular line at the fifth intercostal space. The transcutaneous pacemaker delivers energy through the chest wall to the heart with the aim of depolarizing the heart. These pacemakers can be very uncomfortable for patients as the energy level required is increased to cause capture. Ideal energy levels are between 40 and 60 mA but sometimes a higher energy level is needed to achieve depolarization. Sedation and/ or analgesia should be considered to promote patient comfort.

Clinical Pearls

Transcutaneous Pacemakers

1. When applying pacer pads to the chest, ensure good contact by smoothing the pads on after application to avoid air pockets underneath the pads.
2. Avoid touching the sticky surface of the pads when the energy is being delivered as this can cause microshocks to the provider.

Temporary Transvenous Pacemakers

Temporary transvenous pacemakers (TTVP) are used for short-term pacing. The components of a TTVP include a battery-powered pulse generator and a pacemaker lead (see Figure 5.2). The pacemaker lead is in contact with the endocardium and delivers electrical impulses with the goal of depolarizing the heart.

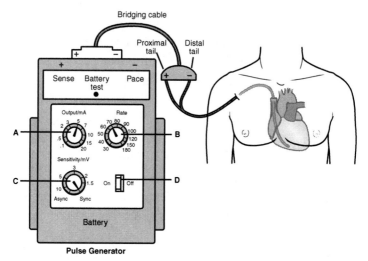

Figure 5.2 ▨ Example of temporary pacemaker.

Clinical Pearls

Temporary Transvenous Pacemakers

1. Ensure the pacer lead posts are securely tightened in the pulse generator.
2. Always have an extra battery (usually 9 V) close at hand in case of battery failure.
3. Observe pacemaker insertion site carefully for redness, inflammation, drainage.
4. Ensure the dressing is intact at pacemaker insertion site.

Single-Chamber Versus Dual-Chamber Pacemakers

The pacemaker lead is most commonly placed in the right ventricle (single chamber) but may also have dual leads with one pacemaker wire in the right atria and one in the right ventricle (dual-chamber or AV sequential pacemaker). In the case of a dual-chamber pacemaker, the impulse may be fired into the atria and then into the ventricle as needed to cause depolarization in one chamber of both with the aim of maximizing cardiac output.

Fixed-Rate Versus Demand Pacing

Pacemakers are programmed to deliver electrical impulses when needed (demand pacemaker) or at a set interval (fixed-rate pacemaker). For example, a demand pacemaker works in the following way: If the pacemaker is programmed for a rate of 70 beats/minute and the intrinsic rate falls below 70 beats/minute, the pacemaker will begin to fire. In contrast, if the pacemaker is programmed with a fixed rate of 70 beats/minute, the pacemaker will deliver impulses at 70 beats/minute regardless of the patient's intrinsic rate.

International Pacemaker Codes

An international pacemaker code provides a universal method of recognizing pacemaker code programming. As a nurse working in a critical care unit, it is most common to refer to the first three letters in the code. All five letters of the code are explained in this section.

The first letter in the code refers to the chamber that is paced. For instance, if the pacemaker is a single-chamber ventricular pacemaker, the code letter will be "V." In contrast, if the pacemaker is a dual-chamber pacer with leads in both the atria and the ventricle, the code would be "D" for dual. Some pacemakers can be turned off for diagnostic reasons and hence have the "O" designation.

The second letter refers to the chamber that is sensed. Sensing only occurs when the pacemaker is a "demand" pacemaker and therefore the code letter would be identified as "V" for ventricle, "A" for atria, or "D" for dual. Should the pacemaker be a fixed-rate pacer, the code would be "O" for none because a fixed-rate pacer does not include a sensing function. For example, a VOO pacemaker would refer to a pacemaker that is paced in the ventricle but there is no sensing or response to sensing function.

The third letter in the pacer code refers to the pacemaker's response to what it has sensed. For example, if the pacemaker senses that the heart's rate has dropped too low, it may trigger ("T") the pacer to fire. Whereas, the inhibit ("I") function refers to the ability of the pacemaker to hold back or inhibit the pacemaker impulse if it senses the heart's own intrinsic activity. The benefit of the sensing function is that it allows for intrinsic activity within the heart and prevents competition between the pacemaker and the intrinsic heart function.

The fourth letter in the code indicates the programmability functions of the pacemaker. It may have no programmability functions, indicated by an "O," however, this is very rare and was primarily seen only in older pacemaker technology. The "P" indicates simple programmable functions versus "M," which indicates a pacemaker that has multiple parameters (e.g., rate, sensing, refractory periods, and output) that can be programmed (often seen in a dual-chamber pacemaker). The "C" indicates that a pacemaker can transmit or receive data for programming purposes. Finally, if the pacemaker has an "R" code in the fourth placement of the letter code, this indicates a rate-responsive function.

Last, the fifth letter of the code indicates antitachyarrhythmia functions. When there is no antitachyarrhythmia function, there will be an "O" designation. "P" refers to the ability to pace and try to recapture a tachycardic rhythm and "S" refers to an ability of the pacer to shock a tachycardia (e.g., ventricular tachycardia or ventricular fibrillation). "D" indicates that there is both a pacing and a shock function that is most commonly seen in an implantable cardiac defibrillator (ICD). For an overview detailing the pacemaker codes, see Table 5.2.

Pacemaker Complications

Pacemaker complications can occur with transcutaneous pacemakers, as well as transvenous and permanent pacemakers. Transcutaneous pacemakers (in which sticky pads/electrodes are

Table 5.2 ▧ *International Pacemaker Codes*

I	II	III	IV	V
Chamber(s) paced	Chamber(s) sensed	Response to sensing	Programmability	Antitachycardic Arrhythmia functions
O–none	O–none	O–none	O–none	O–none
A–atrial	A–atrial	T– trigger	P–simple programmable	P–pacing
V– ventricular	V– ventricular	I–inhibit	M–multi-programmable	S–shock
D–dual (A + V)	D–dual (A + V)	D–both (T + I)	C– communicating	D–dual (P + S)
			R-rate modulation	

Sources: North American Society of Pacing and Electrophysiology/The British Pacing and Electrophysiology Group.

placed on the chest) can result in skin burns, coughing, muscle contractions, pain, and failure to pace. Temporary and permanent pacemakers can result in complications such as air embolus, infection, bleeding, pneumothorax (rare), arrhythmias, hematoma, and perforation of the right ventricle. It is essential to closely monitor the patient's rhythm, vital signs, level of consciousness, presence of chest discomfort, and respiratory status, particularly upon insertion of a temporary transvenous or permanent pacemaker.

Analysis of Pacemaker Strips ... Step by Step

To analyze the pacemaker rhythm strip, *first ensure the patient is stable* and then apply four simple steps.

Step 1: Calculate the pacemaker rate. To do this, measure the number of small squares between two consecutive pacemaker spikes and divide into 1,500. An alternate way to calculate the paced rate is to count the number of pacemaker spikes in a 6-second strip and multiply by 10.

Step 2: Calculate the AV interval. This step only applies to dual-chamber pacemakers. The AV interval is similar to a PR interval but is artificially created by the impulse to the atrium and to the ventricles when the pacemaker is sensed in both chambers (the atria and the ventricle).

Step 3: Observe for intrinsic rhythm. Intrinsic rhythm refers to any underlying rhythm generated by the heart versus by the pacemaker. If the patient is being 100% paced, it would be very difficult to see any intrinsic rhythm.

Step 4: Note any pacemaker malfunction. Analyze the pacemaker rhythm strip to determine whether there are any signs of pacemaker malfunction such as failure to capture, undersensing, or oversensing. Pacemakers are discussed in detail in the next section.

Clinical Pearls

How to Spot Pacemaker Spikes

- Look for small vertical spikes.
- May be difficult to see in all leads.
- Amplitude depends on position and type of lead.
- Bipolar leads result in a much smaller pacing spike than unipolar leads (and bipolar leads are most common).
- Epicardial leads (placed directly on the epicardium) are typically cause smaller spikes than leads that are in contact with the endocardium.
- In atrial pacing, the pacing spike precedes the P wave.
- In a ventricular pacemaker, pacing spikes precede the QRS complex.
- Right ventricle pacing lead placement results in a QRS morphology similar to a premature ventricular contraction.
- Dual-chamber pacemakers may exhibit features of atrial pacing, ventricular pacing, or both.
- In dual-chamber pacing, pacing spikes may precede only the P wave, only the QRS complex, or both depending on the programming and sensing functions.

Examples of Pacemaker Analysis

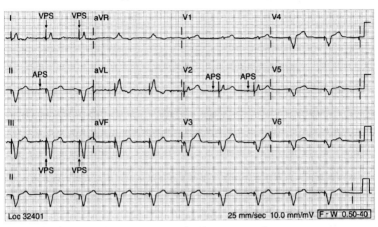

Figure 5.3 ■ Pacemaker strip analysis.

Step 1: Calculate pacemaker rate: rate = 65 (1500/23 small squares = 65)

Step 2: Not a dual chamber pacemaker therefore no AV interval to be calculated

Step 3: No intrinsic rhythm seen since rhythm is 100% paced in this example

Step 4: No pacemaker malfunction seen

Analysis: Ventricular paced rhythm at 65 beats/minute, no intrinsic rhythm seen and no pacemaker malfunction noted.

Pacemaker Malfunction

Three types of pacemaker malfunction (failure to capture, undersensing, and oversensing) are described in the following section.

Failure to Capture

Capture refers to the pacemaker's ability to cause depolarization within the heart. *Failure to capture* refers to the fact that the electrical impulse was discharged but did not cause depolarization (see example in the following section).

The clinical presentation that accompanies failure to capture often includes return of prepacemaker symptoms such as chest discomfort, shortness of breath, hypotension, and weakness. Causes of failure to capture can include milliamperes set too low, medications, poor contact with the endocardium, edema, battery failure, or fracture of the pacing lead. Immediate treatment is required because the patient can deteriorate very quickly with this type of pacemaker malfunction. Emergency treatment includes replacing the battery if needed, turning the patient onto his or her left side in an attempt to increase contact of the pacemaker lead with the endocardium, monitoring vital signs and level of consciousness closely, and calling for assistance.

Capture Versus Failure to Capture

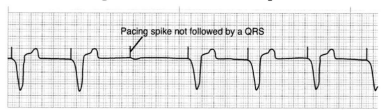

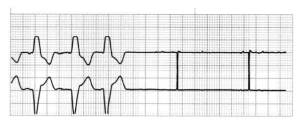

Figure 5.4 ■ Two examples of failure to capture.

Undersensing refers to the pacemaker's inability to sense the heart's intrinsic function (see Figure 5.5). In this situation, the pacemaker does not sense the intrinsic rhythm and fires anyway. The risk of undersensing is that pacemaker spikes will fall randomly onto the heart's intrinsic rhythm and may set up a situation of competition between the pacemaker and the intrinsic rhythm. If the pacemaker impulse is discharged at an inappropriate time, there is a potential for the impulse to hit at a vulnerable period of relative refractoriness (T wave) and cause a lethal arrhythmia such as ventricular fibrillation. Treatment for this malfunction involves adjusting the sensitivity control of the pacemaker. Causes of failure to sense or undersense include battery failure, fracture of pacing lead, edema or fibrosis at catheter tip, and failure of pacemaker circuitry.

Oversensing refers to the pacemaker inhibiting or "holding back" an impulse because it thinks that it is sensing intrinsic heart activity when in fact it is not. The inhibition of the pacemaker impulse results in no impulse being delivered when it should be and a subsequent potential decrease in cardiac output for the patient. Oversensing and the pacemaker not firing can result in the patient becoming very hemodynamically unstable. Causes of oversensing include interference from electromagnetic fields (e.g., welding machines) (see Figure 5.6).

Undersensing (Failure to Sense)

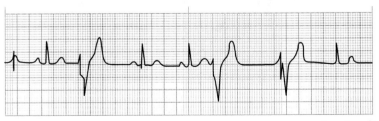

(*continued*)

(continued)

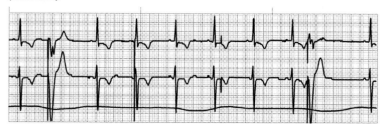

Figure 5.5 ■ Two examples of failure to sense.

Oversensing

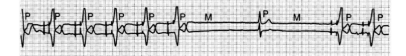

Figure 5.6 ■ Oversensing.

EXERCISES

Case Study

Mrs. W., a 64-year-old female patient, is admitted into the emergency department and states she has been feeling very light-headed and dizzy. Her monitor shows the following:

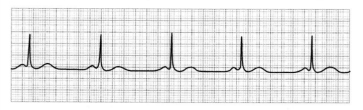

1. This rhythm is _____.

(continued)

(continued)

Her blood pressure (B/P) is 74/42, respiratory rate is 22, O_2 saturation is 95% on room air, and her temperature is 37°C. She begins to lose consciousness and the physician rapidly decides to apply a transcutaneous pacemaker. Her rhythm strip shows the following:

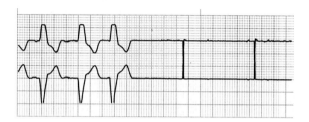

2. Analyze the rhythm on the strip: _____.
3. Priority treatment for this patient includes: _____.
4. If this issue is not resolved what may be a potential alternative?
5. What pacemaker complications must the patient be observed for?

Test Yourself!

1. According to the most recent American Heart Association guidelines (2015), what is the first drug administered in a PEA or asystolic arrest?
   a. Atropine 1 mg
   b. Amiodarone 300 mg
   c. Epinephrine 1 mg

(continued)

(continued)

> **2.** List six potential causes of PEA.
> **3.** Undersensing or failure to sense refers to which of the following?
>> a. The pacemaker's inability to sense the heart's intrinsic function
>> b. The pacemaker inhibits or "holds back" an impulse
>> c. The electrical impulse is discharged but does not cause depolarization
> **4.** A pacemaker that has a DDD code refers to which of the following?
>> a. Paced in the ventricle, sensed in both chambers
>> b. Paced in both the atria and the ventricle
>> c. Has inhibit functions only and does not trigger events

Practice Strips

Systematically interpret each rhythm.

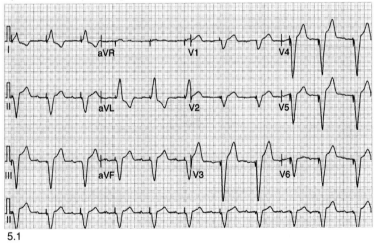

5.1

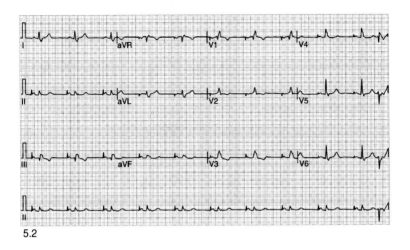

5.2

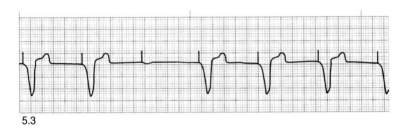

5.3

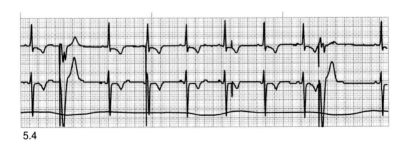

5.4

(See answers for Chapter 5 in the "Answers" chapter.)

RESOURCES

Aehlert, B. (2013). *ECGs made easy* (5th ed.). St. Louis, MO: Mosby.

American Heart Association. (2015). 2015 American Heart Association guidelines for cardiopulmonary resuscitation and emergency cardiac care. *Circulation, 132*(18, Suppl. 2), s313–s573. doi:10.1161/cir.00000000000261

Goldsworthy, S. (2012). *Coronary care 1 and 2 manual.* Oshawa, ON: Durham College Continuing Education.

International pacemaker codes. (2015). Retrieved from www .pacemaker.vuuwerl.nl/info/nbg_code_naspe.htm

Walraven, G. (2011). *Basic arrhythmias* (7th ed.). Toronto, ON: Pearson.

6

12-Lead EKG Overview

This chapter presents an overview of 12-lead EKG interpretation. Here, practical clinical tips are provided that will assist you in obtaining the best possible tracing and guide you through a step-by-step approach to 12-lead EKG interpretation. In addition, 15-lead EKGs are discussed. The chapter concludes with practice questions and a case study you can use to assess your retention of the information discussed here.

Although 12-lead EKG interpretation and diagnosis falls within the scope of medicine, our role as critical care nurses is essential in the early recognition and assessment of the patient when subtle (or not so subtle!) changes occur on the EKG. As is often said, "time is muscle" when ischemia and injury are occurring within the myocardium. The sooner EKG changes and deterioration in patient status are noted; the sooner treatment can be implemented with the goal of optimizing the outcome for the patient.

THE BASICS

Because the heart is a three-dimensional organ, 12-lead EKGs provide us with 12 different leads or "views" of the heart from different angles. When a patient has experienced a myocardial infarction (MI), this view of the heart is particularly helpful in determining which face(s) of the heart was involved (e.g., lateral, anterior, posterior, or inferior). By placing six precordial (chest) electrodes and four limb electrodes, we are able to generate 12 different views of the heart on the EKG.

The six limb leads (aVL, aVR, aVF, I, II, III) view the heart in a vertical plane (up and down) called the frontal plane. The frontal plane can be imagined as a circle superimposed on the patient's body. Imagine holding a hula hoop in front of you against your body. If you marked off the circle or hula hoop in degrees, this would represent the limb leads view of electrical forces (depolarization and repolarization) moving up and down and left and right on a frontal plane. Each lead has its own angle of orientation or view of the heart. This angle is expressed in circle. See Table 6.1 for the angle of orientation of the three standard limb leads (I, II, and III) and also for the three augmented limb leads (aVR, aVL, aVF).

Table 6.1 ▪ *Limb Lead Description*

Lead	Description
I	Created by making the left arm positive and the right arm negative. Angle of orientation = 0°
II	Created by making the legs positive and the right arm negative. Angle of orientation = +60°

(continued)

Table 6.1 ■ *Limb Lead Description (continued)*

Lead	Description
III	Created by making the legs positive and the right arm negative. Angle of orientation = +120°
aVL	Created by making the left arm positive and the other limbs negative. Angle of orientation = -30°
aVR	Created by making the right arm positive and the other limbs negative. Angle of orientation = -150°
aVF	Is created by making the legs positive and the other limbs negative. Angle of orientation = +90°
Putting it all together	

Source: www.nataliescasebook.com

PRECORDIAL LEADS

The precordial or chest leads record electrical forces moving anteriorly and posteriorly through the chest and are referred to as V1, V2, V3, V4, V5, and V6.

PROPER LEAD PLACEMENT

Proper lead placement is important in assessing for changes on the EKG over time. The six chest electrodes are placed on the chest in the configuration shown in Table 6.2. In addition, an electrode is placed on the fleshy part of each limb.

Table 6.2 ■ *Precordial Leads*

Lead	Placement
V1	Fourth intercostal space to right of sternum
V2	Fourth intercostal space to left of sternum
V3	Between V3 and V4
V4	Fifth intercostal space midclavicular line
V5	Between V4 and V6
V6	Fifth intercostal space midaxillary line
Putting it all together	

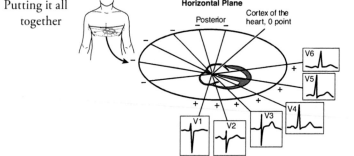

Source: www.publicsafety.net

Clinical Pearls

Tips for Obtaining the Best Tracings

In order to obtain the best tracings on the EKG, here are a few practical tips:

■ Avoid placing electrodes over bony prominences, aim for the fleshy part of the distal limb for limb leads.

(continued)

(continued)

- ▓ Electrodes can dry out over time and may need to be replaced for the best tracing.
- ▓ The patient needs to be as still as possible to obtain the best tracing.
- ▓ In the patient's room, avoid multiple plug-ins of electrical equipment wherever possible, this can sometimes cause electrical interference and difficulty reading the EKG.
- ▓ Prepare the skin with skin-prep pads and make sure the skin is dry. Occasionally, skin may need to be shaved to improve direct contact of the electrode with the skin.

INDICATIONS

A 12-lead EKG is indicated for several reasons, such as suspected MI, angina, and arrhythmias. The EKG can also provide information about electrolyte imbalance and clinical conditions such as pericarditis and chronic obstructive pulmonary disease (COPD). It is a diagnostic test that can be quickly completed and is noninvasive.

STEP-BY-STEP APPROACH TO 12-LEAD EKG INTERPRETATION

The following step-by-step approach is recommended as a systematic way to analyze the findings of your patient's EKG. Prior to conducting this analysis, it is always important to assess the patient's status first and then proceed to the analysis of the EKG.

Step 1: Analyze the rhythm. Generally, you will look at lead II to do this and often there is a longer strip of lead II present at the bottom of the 12-lead EKG that can be used for this purpose. Utilize the systematic approach to interpreting arrhythmias outlined in Chapter 2 of this book to assist you with your approach to this step.

Step 2: Analyze the axis. *Axis* refers to the average direction of electrical flow in the heart. To get started with analyzing axis, look at aVF and lead I on the EKG. aVF and lead I should both be upright or mostly positive (above the isoelectric line or baseline). If they are both upright, this indicates a normal axis deviation (NAD; Table 6.3).

Table 6.3 ▪ *Axis Determination*

Axis	aVF	Lead I	Potential Causes
Normal axis deviation	Positive	Positive	Normal
Left axis deviation	Negative	Positive	Obesity Pregnancy Left bundle branch block (LBBB) Inferior MI Wolf–Parkinson–White syndrome (WPW)
Right axis deviation	Positive	Negative	Lateral MI Right bundle branch block (RBBB) Right ventricular hypertrophy Acute lung disease Hyperkalemia Can be normal in children and tall, thin adults
Extreme right axis deviation ("no-man's land")	Negative	Negative	Pacing Ventricular tachycardia

Step 3: R wave progression and transition. Step 3 involves assessing the R waves for progression. Specifically, the R wave should become larger in amplitude as it moves from V1 to V6. Commonly, V5 is the largest R wave and V6 slightly smaller

because V5 is closest to the apex of the heart. Part of observing the R wave progression is noting where "transition" occurs. *Transition* refers to the point at which the R wave and the S wave are most equiphasic (one half below the isoelectric line and one half above the isoelectric line). Causes of loss of R wave progression include left ventricular hypertrophy and an anterior MI.

Step 4: Assess voltage. When assessing voltage across the 12-lead EKG, the QRS amplitude in the limb leads (I, II, II, aVF, aVL, aVR), need to be greater than 5 mm (five small squares or one large square in total height). Remember to count the S wave in the height as well (not just the R wave). When assessing the precordial leads, V1 to V6, the QRS voltage should be greater than 10 mm (at least 10 small squares or two large squares). Should the voltage fall below these parameters in two contiguous leads (two or more in limb leads or two or more in the precordial leads), then the voltage is classified as low. Causes of low voltage include factors such as barrel chest, pericardial effusion, poor lead contact, and subcutaneous emphysema. Causes of increased voltage include ventricular hypertrophy, which is discussed in Step 6 (Table 6.4).

Table 6.4 ■ *Summary of Voltage Assessment*

Limb leads (I, II, III, aVL, aVR, aVF)	QRS amplitude needs to be > 5 mm If < 5 mm in two or more limb leads = low voltage
Precordial leads (V1–V6)	QRS amplitude needs to be > 10 mm If < 10 mm in two or more precordial leads = low voltage

Step 5: Assess for bundle branch block. In Step 5, you will be assessing whether a left bundle branch block (LBBB) or a right bundle branch block (RBBB) is present. If you have determined that the EKG is of normal duration in Step 1, you can confidently say there is no bundle branch block (BBB) and move on to Step 5. If, however, the QRS was found to be more

than 0.12 seconds, further assessment is required. A BBB refers to the fact that conduction is proceeding in a delayed fashion down the right bundle pathway or the left bundle pathway, thereby delaying the conduction velocity and causing the QRS to be widened (> 0.12 seconds). See Table 6.5 for causes, characteristics, and treatment of LBBB and RBBB.

Table 6.5 ▪ *Left and Right Bundle Branch Blocks*

	Left Bundle Branch Block	*Right Bundle Branch Block*
Causes	▪ Conduction delay in the left bundle branch ▪ Usually happens as a consequence of other diseases such as arteriosclerosis, rheumatic heart disease, myocarditis, congenital heart disease, MI, metastatic heart tumors, or other invasions of the heart tissue	▪ Conduction delay in the right bundle branch ▪ Right ventricular hypertrophy/cor pulmonale ▪ Pulmonary embolism ▪ Ischemic heart disease ▪ Congenital heart disease ▪ Myocarditis
Characteristics	▪ Rhythm, rate, P wave, PR interval (PRi) normal ▪ QRS > 0.12 seconds ▪ ST usually abnormal in size and configuration—occurs in opposite direction of QRS ▪ T wave opposite to QRS in most leads ▪ I, aVL, V5, and V6 broad on top or notched QRS ▪ Left axis deviation may be present	▪ Rate, rhythm, PRi normal ▪ QRS > 0.12 seconds ▪ ST and T waves opposite of QRS ▪ RSR[1] in V1 and V2 with ST depression and T wave inversion ▪ I, aVL, V5, V6 all have deep S wave

(continued)

Table 6.5 ■ *Left and Right Bundle Branch Blocks (continued)*

	Left Bundle Branch Block	Right Bundle Branch Block
Treatment	■ Treat the underlying cause	
EKG	Left bundle branch block characteristics	Right bundle branch block characteristics

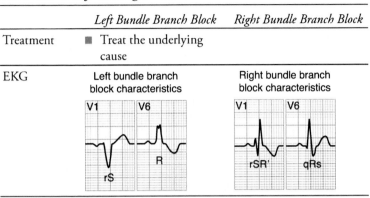

MI, myocardial infarction.

Note: An MI cannot be diagnosed on the 12-lead EKG alone with the presence of a new left bundle branch block.

Step 6: Assess for hypertrophy. Step 6 involves assessing for atrial and ventricular hypertrophy. Although the 12-lead EKG can provide some information about hypertrophy, other diagnostic tests, such as echocardiography, can provide us with a more accurate clinical picture. Table 6.6 provides a summary of causes and characteristics of hypertrophy as it is displayed on the EKG.

Table 6.6 ■ *Hypertrophy on the 12-Lead EKG*

Hypertrophy	Potential Causes	Characteristics
Left atrial hypertrophy	Mitral stenosis	■ Tall (> 3 mm) *peaked* P wave in lead II
Right atrial hypertrophy	Chronic lung disease Tricuspid stenosis Congenital heart disease Pulmonary hypertension	■ Wide (0.11 seconds) notched p (m-shaped) in lead II

(continued)

Table 6.6 ▨ *Hypertrophy on the 12-Lead EKG (continued)*

Hypertrophy	Potential Causes	Characteristics
Left ventricular hypertrophy	Hypertension Aortic valve stenosis Normal in conditioned athletes Hypertrophic cardiomyopathy	▨ Use precordial leads, look for very *large amplitude of QRS* (e.g., R wave amplitude in V5 and V6 plus the S wave amplitude in V1 and V2 > 35 mm)
Right ventricular hypertrophy	Pulmonary hypertension Pulmonic valve stenosis Emphysema Pulmonary embolus	▨ R wave larger than S in V1 and V2 ▨ S wave larger than R in V5 and V6 ▨ Right axis deviation ▨ Possible right atrial enlargement ▨ ST–T wave V1 and V2 show RV strain pattern

Step 7: Is there an MI? Perhaps one of the most critical steps in analyzing the 12-lead EKG is the assessment of the 12 views for the presence of an MI or ischemia. In order to begin this step, I suggest that you systematically look at each "face" of the heart (i.e., anterior, lateral, posterior, and inferior). Groupings of specific leads provide information about each "face" or side of the heart. For instance: Lead II, III, and aVF together look at the inferior side of the heart and can provide information about the presence of an inferior MI. Leads V3 and V4 look most directly at the anterior surface of the heart and provide information about the possibility that the patient might be having an anterior MI or ischemia in this area. Lateral MIs can be assessed by analyzing the lateral leads,

which are I, aVL, V5, and V6. Finally, the posterior portion of the heart is best assessed by performing a 15-lead EKG. The 15-lead EKG can also provide information related to whether the patient is experiencing a right ventricular MI. Practical tips on performing a 15-lead EKG are provided in the following section.

Clinical Pearls	**Where to Search for MIs on the 12-Lead EKG**

Anterior MI	Lateral MI	Inferior MI	Posterior MI	RV MI
V3 V4	I aVL, V5, and V6	II, III, aVF	V8, V9 (on 15 lead)	V4R (on 15 lead)

To assess for potential ischemic or infarction changes, start with one face of the heart (e.g., anterior) and note any ST segment and/or T wave changes. Specifically observe for ST depression (represents ischemic changes) or ST elevation (injury—usually indicating an MI) above the isoelectric or baseline. Should you notice any of these changes across the 12-lead EKG, it is imperative that you notify the most responsible physician immediately because, as mentioned previously, "time is muscle." The sooner treatment is initiated, the better the outcome for the patient may be. It is *urgent* that you notify the team of these changes as soon as possible (i.e., stat!). Even a slight elevation or depression of the ST segment is critical. In terms of the T wave, you are assessing to make sure that the T wave is upright and symmetrical, which is normal. If the T wave becomes inverted, this could signal myocardial ischemia.

The second component to assess for ST and T wave changes is to determine the stage of the MI. Initially, when someone is

> *Clinical Pearls*
>
> **Summary of 12-Lead EKG Interpretation**
>
> *Step 1:* Analyze the rhythm
>
> *Step 2:* Analyze the axis
>
> *Step 3:* R wave progression and transition
>
> *Step 4:* Assess voltage
>
> *Step 5:* Assess for bundle branch block
>
> *Step 6:* Assess for hypertrophy
>
> *Step 7:* Is there an MI?

experiencing an MI, the T wave becomes peaked, followed by ST elevation (minutes to hours), T wave inversion, and the appearance of a pathological Q wave (hours to days). This type of an MI is referred to as an ST elevated MI (STEMI), which indicates that the necrosis has proceeded through all three layers of the heart (full-thickness or transmural MI). Some patients experience an infarct or death of tissue in only one layer of the heart; this is referred to as a non-ST elevated MI (NSTEMI). In this type of MI, a pathological Q wave does not typically appear. As the heart reperfuses after treatment, the ST will gradually come back to baseline, the T wave will become upright, and the only part that will remain is the pathological Q wave (in a STEMI). It is also important to note that the 12-lead EKG is not typically used in isolation to diagnose an MI, but rather the combination of cardiac markers, history, and a 12-lead EKG are the gold standard in initially diagnosing an MI. The MI proceeds through stages usually identified as the hyperacute phase (ST elevation), acute phase (ST elevation), T wave inversion and Q waves starting to appear, and old or resolved phase with only the pathological Q wave remaining (Table 6.7).

Table 6.7 ▪ *Abnormal Waves in a Myocardial Infarction: ST,*
Q Wave, and Inverted T Waves

Waveform	Important Notes
Abnormal Q wave	▪ The appearance of a new Q wave signals infarction
	▪ Usually appear within several hours of the onset of infarction
	▪ > 0.04 seconds and/or deeper than one third the height of the R wave
	▪ Note: Small Q waves are normal in some leads: I, aVL, V5, and V6, and sometimes II and III
ST elevation or depression	▪ ST elevation signals injury
	▪ ST depression signals ischemia
	▪ Pathological ST elevation typically presents with a bowed upward configuration ("tombstone")
T waves	▪ Usually peak initially and within hours become inverted
	▪ T wave inversion signals ischemia
	▪ Can be seen in angina and myocardial infarction
	▪ Pathological T wave inversion occurs symmetrically versus asymmetrically or "sloping"

THE NORMAL 12-LEAD EKG

Before we move on to the abnormal EKG it is important to be familiar with the normal EKG. Use the step-by-step approach described previously to apply the 12-lead EKG seen in Figure 6.1. You will find that all parameters are within the normal range. For instance, the axis is normal, R wave progression is normal, transition occurs at V3 or V4, there is no hypertrophy, no BBB, and no MI present (as evidenced by no abnormal ST and T wave changes).

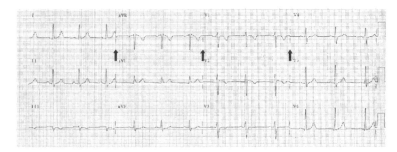

Figure 6.1 ■ Normal 12-lead EKG.

15-LEAD EKGs

The 15-lead EKG allows us to gather information about whether a right ventricular MI and/or a posterior MI might be present. To obtain a 15-lead EKG we simply remove V4 and move it over to the same position on the right side of the chest and label it V4R, we then remove V5 and V6 and move them into the V8 and V9 positions to enable us to view the heart directly from the posterior side. V8 should be placed at the fifth intercostal space midscapular line and V9 should be placed between V8 and the spine.

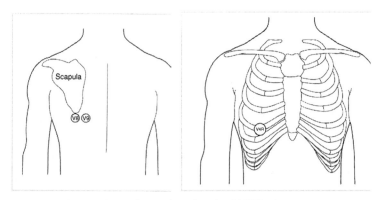

Figure 6.2 ■ Examples of 15-lead EKG placement.

EXERCISES

Mr. J., 66 years old, appears in the emergency department at 2 a.m. and states that he has had pressure in the center of his chest for the last hour and has felt very weak and nauseous. He has a history of type 2 diabetes for the past 15 years and also smokes one package of cigarettes per day. His vital signs on admission are:

Pulse: 56/min/regular
Blood pressure (B/P): 96/52
Respiratory rate: 20/min
O_2 saturation: 95% on room air

He is placed on a cardiac monitor, a left peripheral intravenous line is started to keep vein open (TKVO) and bloodwork is drawn for cardiac markers, complete blood count, and electrolytes

An EKG is performed (see the following) and nitro spray is administered.

1. Using the step-by-step approach to interpreting 12-lead EKGs (from this chapter) interpret his 12-lead EKG in the following.

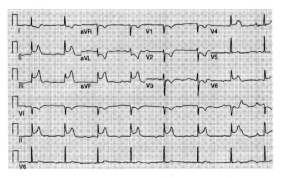

1. Myocardial injury appears on the EKG as:
   a. T wave inversion alone
   b. ST segment elevation
   c. Pathological Q waves
   d. PR interval lengthening

2. Which leads look most directly at the anterior surface of the left ventricle?
   a. I, II, III
   b. I, aVL
   c. V3, V4
   d. aVR, aVL

3. A 45-year-old man was admitted to the emergency department with severe chest pain. He rated the pain as a 10 on a scale of 1–10. He is ashen and diaphoretic. His 12-lead shows hyperacute ST segments in II, III, and aVF. He is most likely suffering from:
   a. Stable angina
   b. An acute inferior infarct
   c. An acute anterior infarct
   d. A chronic lateral infarct

4. These characteristics describe the following: RSR[1] in leads V1 and V2, QRS > 0.12 seconds:
   a. RBBB
   b. LBBB
   c. Right anterior hemiblock
   d. There is no abnormality

(See answers for Chapter 6 in the "Answers" chapter.)

RESOURCES

Aehlert, B. (2013). *ECGs made easy* (5th ed.). St. Louis, MO: Mosby.

Goldsworthy, S. (2012). *Coronary care II manual*. Oshawa, Canada: Durham College.

Thaler, M. (2012). *The only ECG book you will ever need* (7th ed.). Philadelphia, PA: Wolters Kluwer.

7

Special Situations

OBJECTIVES

In this chapter, several special clinical situations related to the 12-lead EKG are described. The influence of electrolytes, pericarditis, hypothermia, chronic obstructive pulmonary disease (COPD), pulmonary embolism, as well as pharmacological and neurological impact are also explored. Practical tips are provided that offer assistance in recognizing specific pathophysiology and the influence on the electrical functioning of the heart.

SPECIAL SITUATIONS

Pericarditis

Pericarditis involves an inflammation of the pericardium that can be caused by such factors as myocardial infarction (MI), trauma, cardiac surgery, infection, and lupus. The patient often presents with sharp, stabbing substernal pain that exacerbates on inspiration, coughing, and movement. Patients who are experiencing pericarditis usually have a sudden onset of pain that can last for days; some relief of the pain may occur when he or she sits up or leans forward. On assessment, patients with pericarditis present with tachycardia, fever, and pericardial friction rub. Lab values show leukocytosis and an increased sedimentation rate. Usual treatment for pericarditis involves nonsteroidal anti-inflammatory drugs.

EKG Changes

EKG changes in pericarditis include ST elevation and T wave inversion (T waves invert only after ST returns to baseline, unlike an MI). Typically, ST segments are normal in the precordial leads (V1–V6) and aVR but are elevated in other leads. Because of the elevated ST segment, the findings can easily be confused with an MI. In pericarditis, however, there is diffuse ST elevation (concave) present and Q waves do not develop. Other EKG changes include low QRS voltage and depression of the PR interval in limb leads if pericardial effusion is present.

Myocarditis

Myocarditis refers to a diffuse inflammation of the myocardium in the absence of ischemia and is often associated with pericarditis. Common causes include viruses (e.g., coxsackie B, HIV, influenza A), bacteria (mycoplasma, rickettsia, and leptospira), immune-mediated disease (e.g., Kawasaki's disease, lupus, and sarcoidosis), and drugs (e.g., amphetamines). Patients may present with mild chest pain, fever, chills, diaphoresis, and flu-like symptoms.

EKG Changes

Patients experiencing myocarditis can present with bundle branch blocks or hemiblocks on the EKG. Arrhythmias can result and subsequent heart failure, cardiogenic shock, and death may occur in the acute stage. Most common, myocarditis is benign without serious long-term effects. In addition, patient's present with sinus tachycardia, QRS/QT prolongation, diffuse T wave inversion, ventricular arrhythmias, and occasionally atrioventricular (AV) blocks. In rare cases delayed cardiomyopathy may develop. Common causes include viruses (e.g., coxsackie B, HIV, and influenza A), bacteria (mycoplasma, rickettsia, and leptospira), immune-mediated disease (e.g., Kawasaki's disease, lupus, and sarcoidosis), and drugs (e.g., amphetamines).

ELECTROLYTES AND THE EKG—SERUM POTASSIUM AND THE HEART

Hyperkalemia

Patients presenting with increased potassium levels often present with nausea, vomiting, abdominal cramping, weakness, and numbness of the extremities. Causes of hyperkalemia include decreased potassium excretion (e.g., renal disease, adrenal insufficiency, angiotensin-converting enzyme [ACE] inhibitors, and cyclosporine), increased potassium intake (e.g., transfusion of banked blood, potassium penicillin), crush injuries (e.g., rhabdomyolysis, trauma), lysis of cells (e.g., chemotherapy), acidosis, and malignant hyperthermia.

EKG Changes

EKG changes in the patient with hyperkalemia include tall, narrow, peaked T waves and a shortened QT interval. With potassium levels greater than 6 to 7 mEq/L, there is a gradual flattening of P waves; with potassium levels greater than 7 mEq/L, further widening of the QRS is seen, and arryhthmias, such as idioventricular rhythm and asystole, emerge.

Hypokalemia

Patients who are hypokalemic (K < 3.5 mEq/L) typically present with dizziness, muscle cramps, fatigue, orthostatic hypotension, decreased bowel sounds, irritability, and confusion. Causes of hypokalemia include poor potassium intake (e.g., starvation, alcoholism), increased gastrointestinal losses (e.g., gastrointestinal surgery, vomiting, diarrhea, laxative abuse), increased renal losses (e.g., polyuria, sodium restriction, heart failure, cirrhosis, hypomagnesemia), burns, drugs (loop diuretics—furosemide), alkalosis, and profound diaphoresis.

EKG Changes

Hypokalemia presents on the EKG with flat T waves, U waves, and, occasionally, a depressed ST segment. In addition, prolonged QT and PR intervals may be seen. These changes, along with further decreased levels of potassium, can result in dysrhythmias, premature ventricular contractions (PVCs), ventricular tachycardia, ventricular fibrillation, and torsade de pointes.

OTHER ELECTROLYTES (SODIUM, MAGNESIUM, AND CALCIUM) AND THE HEART

Hyponatremia

Signs of decreased levels of sodium include anorexia, nausea, vomiting, headache, generalized weakness, postural hypotension, weight loss, muscle cramps, tremors, and seizures. Causes of hyponatremia include decreased sodium intake (e.g., sodium-restricted diet, alcoholism) and increased sodium excretion (e.g., diaphoresis, burns, gastrointestinal losses, diarrhea, laxative abuse, diuretics, and Addison's disease).

EKG Changes

EKG changes in hyponatremia include sinus tachycardia.

Hypernatremia

High levels of serum sodium, or hypernatremia, are caused by factors such as excess salt consumption, heart failure, renal failure, cirrhosis, Cushing's syndrome, and steroid therapy. Patients experiencing hypernatremia present with thirst, muscle weakness, cramps, hypertension, edema, flushed dry skin, irritability, restlessness, seizures, confusion, weight gain, and oliguria.

EKG Changes

EKG changes in hypernatremia include sinus tachycardia.

Hypocalcemia

Patients presenting with hypoglycemia can experience abdominal cramps, muscle cramps, numbness of fingertips, numbness of circumoral area, and facial twitching in response to facial nerve tapping. In addition, patients with hypoglycemia can present with Trousseau's sign, irritability, seizures, oliguria, or anuria. Causes of hypocalcemia include decreased calcium intake or absorption (e.g., insufficient dietary intake, hypoparathyroidism, hypomagnesemia, renal failure, vitamin D deficiency, liver disease, alcoholism, Cushing's syndrome, and steroid therapy), increased calcium excretion (e.g., use of diuretics, chronic diarrhea, hyperphosphatemia), and increased calcium binding (e.g., acute pancreatitis, alkalosis, heparin, theophylline, cimetidine).

EKG Changes

EKG changes to monitor for in the face of hypocalcemia include prolonged QT intervals and torsades de pointes.

Hypercalcemia

Hypercalcemia can occur as a result of increased calcium intake (e.g., excessive use of calcium supplements), increased calcium absorption (e.g., hypophosphatemia), increased mobilization of calcium from the bone (e.g., hyperparathyroidism, vitamin D excess, immobility, malignancy, thyrotoxicosis), decreased calcium excretion (e.g., Addison's disease). On assessment, patients with hypercalcemia present with thirst, anorexia, nausea, vomiting, abdominal pain, and bone or flank pain. In addition, patients may have decreased bowel sounds, muscular weakness, confusion, renal calculi, azotemia, and polyuria.

EKG Changes

Patients with high levels of calcium can present with shortened QT interval, arrhythmias, and AV blocks.

Hypomagnesemia

Low levels of magnesium, or hypomagmesemia, can be caused by decreased magnesium intake (e.g., malnutrition), impaired absorption (e.g., alcoholism, acute pancreatitis), increased magnesium loss (e.g., diuretics, cyclosporine), vomiting, chronic diarrhea, gastrointestinal suction, diabetic ketoacidosis, and heart failure. On assessment, patients with low magnesium levels can present with anorexia, nausea, vomiting, muscle cramps, syncope, hypotension, seizures, and confusion.

EKG Changes

Patients experiencing hypomagnesemia can present with prolonged QT intervals and dysrhythmias such as sinus tachycardia and torsades de pointes.

Hypermagnesemia

Causes of hypermagnesemia include increased magnesium intake (e.g., magnesium-rich antacids, laxatives, or enemas), decreased magnesium excretion (e.g., renal failure, hyperparathyroidism, hypothyroidism, burns, and rhabdomyolysis). On assessment, patients with high levels of magnesium can present with muscle weakness, fatigue, nausea and vomiting, somnolence, diplopia, hypotension, facial flushing, and confusion. High levels of magnesium can also precipitate cardiac arrest.

EKG Changes

EKG changes in hypermagnesemia include prolonged PR, QRS, and QT intervals. In addition, the patient can develop AV blocks and bradycardia.

ADDITIONAL SITUATIONS TO CONSIDER

Hypothermia

Hypothermia is defined as a core body temperature of less than 35°C. Hypothermia can result from exposure (e.g., near drowning, prolonged exposure to cold temperatures), perioperative hypothermia, or therapeutic hypothermia (e.g., postarrest).

EKG Changes

Arrhythmias that can develop in hypothermia include sinus bradycardia, atrial fibrillation with a slow ventricular response, AV blocks, and junctional rhythms. Ventricular ectopy can emerge as PVCs and progress to ventricular tachycardia and ventricular fibrillation. When the core body temperature dips to 30°C and below, Osborn (J) waves can result. The Osborn wave is a positive deflection at the J point; the height of the Osborn wave is proportional to the degree of hypothermia.

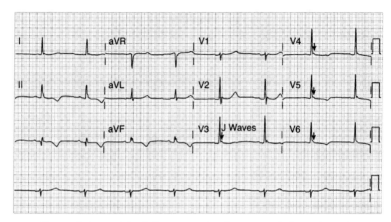

Figure 7.1 ▪ 12-lead demonstrating J waves as in hypothermia.

A shivering artifact can also be seen on the EKG and appears as a fuzzy baseline.

Subarachnoid Bleeds

Subarachnoid hemorrhage can occur as a result of a blunt or penetrating injury to the head, which causes bleeding into the subarachnoid space. Patients present with headache, changes in level of consciousness, nuchal rigidity, and Kernig's sign (inability to extend leg when thigh is flexed on the abdomen).

EKG Changes

EKG changes in a subarachnoid bleed include diffuse T wave inversion, prominent U waves, and sinus bradycardia. In addition, an increasing systolic blood pressure can occur with a widening pulse pressure. Arrhythmias can emerge as a result of circulating catecholamines.

Chronic Obstructive Pulmonary Disease
EKG Changes

EKG changes seen in COPD can include right ventricular hypertrophy, right atrial enlargement, and right axis deviation (which can lead to right ventricular failure). There may be a complete absence of R waves in leads I, II, and III, which results in a deep S wave (RS pattern). In addition, multifocal atrial tachycardia may be seen. Low voltage may be seen as a result of the dampening effect caused by the air trapped in the alveoli.

Pulmonary Embolism

Pulmonary embolism can result from obstruction of one or more arteries of the lung caused by fat, air, blood, or amniotic fluid. In addition, a pulmonary embolism could result from a tumor or foreign body. Pulmonary embolism risk factors include fracture of the long bones (fat embolism), venous stasis (e.g., prolonged bedrest, air travel), surgical procedures (air embolus), hypercoagulability (e.g., malignancy, dehydration), or trauma to the vessel wall. On assessment, the patient is often anxious, dyspneic, tachypneic, tachycardic, and experiencing chest pain. In addition, troponin I levels may be elevated as a result of right ventricular microinfarction.

EKG Changes

When a pulmonary embolism is present, the EKG can display right ventricular hypertrophy, right bundle branch block (RBBB), tall peaked P waves, a large S wave in V1, and a deep Q wave in lead III. Sinus tachycardia and atrial fibrillation may present in the face of a pulmonary embolism.

Hypothyroidism

Causes of hypothyroidism can include Hashimoto's thyroiditis, surgical removal of the thyroid gland, drugs (e.g., lithium and amiodarone), and pituitary disease. Patients with hypothyroidism may present with hypothermia, hypotension, hyponatremia, hypoglycemia, and lethargy that can progress to coma.

EKG Changes

Hypothyroidism can cause ST depression and bradycardia. In addition, the patient may have prolonged conduction times, prominent T waves, and T wave inversion. Left ventricular hypertrophy may also be present.

Trauma (Myocardial)

The severity of trauma to the chest can vary. *Commotio cordis* refers to sudden cardiac death from a blow to the anterior chest (e.g., hockey puck or baseball). Other blunt trauma to the chest can cause myocardial contusion resulting in arrhythmias and tachycardia. If the trauma has caused valve damage or disruption, a heart murmur can result. Other results of trauma to the chest can result in pericardial effusion and tamponade. Patients experiencing trauma to the chest are typically monitored for at least 24 hours in hospital for sudden emergence of arrhythmias and/or for surgical intervention.

EKG Changes

When there has been trauma to the chest, the EKG can display nonspecific ST and T wave changes. In addition, the patient has a high risk of arrhythmia and AV node blocks.

Clinical Pearls

QT Monitoring: When to Monitor and Who Is at Risk?

Why monitor QT intervals?

The risk of a prolonged QT interval is that the next impulse could strike the vulnerable portion of the T wave just before the heart is ready to accept another impulse; should this happen *ventricular fibrillation can occur*. This is referred to as the R-on-T phenomenon.

Who Is at Risk?

- Congenital prolonged QT
- Significant bradycardia
- Antidysrhytmics such as quinidine, procainamide, sotalol
- Electrolyte imbalances: especially hypokalemia, hypomagnesemia, hypocalcemia
- Drugs: tricyclic antidepressants (e.g., Elavil), erythromycin
- Hypothermia
- Hypothyroidism
- Hypoglycemia
- Myocardial infarction
- Heart failure

FINAL THOUGHTS … SUMMARY

In this compact clinical guide, systematic approaches have been provided to assist you in interpreting basic rhythms and for approaching a 12-lead EKG. Special situations related to the 12-lead EKG have been identified in this chapter, with practical tips on how to recognize specific clinical conditions and the impact this pathophysiology may have on the EKG. To ensure your ongoing competence and confidence in the area of arrhythmia interpretation and 12-lead EKG analysis, I encourage you to continue to review these principles and approaches as well as to attend ongoing professional development opportunities such as grand rounds, workshops, and major conferences.

EXERCISES

Case Study

Mrs. W., a 50-year-old female patient, arrives in the emergency department and states she has had a prolonged period of persistent diarrhea. She has poor skin turgor and has moderate ascites. Her vital signs are:

Heart rate (HR): 118 beats/minute
Blood pressure (B/P): 84/46
Respiratory rate: 22
O_2 saturation: 95% on room air
Temperature: 37.9°C

She states her muscles have been very "crampy." She has a long history of alcoholism and states she does not have much appetite. As you are assessing her, she suddenly loses consciousness and reverts from sinus tachycardia to the rhythm seen here.

1. Identify your priority actions.
2. What is this rhythm called?
3. What do you suspect has caused this rhythm to occur?

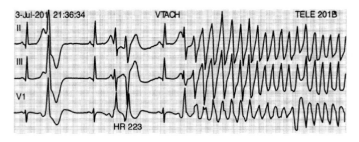

3-Jul-201 21:36:34   VTACH   TELE 201B

II

III

V1

HR 223

> ### Test Yourself!
>
> **1.** What is the risk of a prolonged QT interval?
> **2.** Differentiate between hyperkalemia and hypokalemia on the EKG.
> **3.** Subarachnoid bleeds can often cause which arrhythmia?
>   a. Sinus tachycardia
>   b. Atrial fibrillation
>   c. Sinus bradycardia
>   d. Junctional rhythms
> **4.** Osborne waves are seen in which of the following conditions?
>   a. Hypothermia
>   b. Myocarditis
>   c. Cardiac contusion
>   d. Pulmonary embolus

(See answers for Chapter 7 in the "Answers" chapter.)

RESOURCES

American Heart Association. (2015). 2015 American Heart Association guidelines for cardiopulmonary resuscitation and emergency cardiac care. *Circulation*, *132*(18, Suppl. 2), s313–s573. American Heart Association, doi:10.1161/cir.00000000000261

Baird, M. (2015). *Manual of critical care nursing: Nursing interventions and collaborative management.* St. Louis, MO: Elsevier.

Dennison, R. (2013). *Pass CCRN!* (4th ed.). St. Louis, MO: Elsevier.

Merck Manual (professional edition). (2015). Retrieved from http://www.merckmanuals.com/professional/injuries-poisoning/thoracic-trauma/blunt-cardiac-injury

Pagana, K., & Pagana, T. (2014). *Mosby's handbook of laboratory and diagnostic tests* (5th ed.). St. Louis, MO: Elsevier.

Thaler, M. (2012). *The only ECG book you will ever need* (7th ed.). Philadelphia, PA: Wolters Kluwer.

Answers

Chapter 1

Test Yourself!

1. Factors that affect stroke volume are preload, afterload, and contractility.
2. Inotropic factors are those factors that impact contractility. A positive inotrope increases contractility, whereas a negative inotrope decreases contractility.
3. P wave = atrial depolarization

   QRS = ventricular depolarization

   T wave = ventricular repolarization

   QT interval = time it takes the ventricles to depolarize and repolarize
4. a
5. a
6. The normal conduction pathway in the heart is: SA node–>internodal branches–>AV node–>bundle of HIS–> bundle branches and purkinje fibers.

Chapter 2

Case Study

1. Stable (symptomatic but maintaining blood pressure and level of consciousness)
2. Supraventricular tachycardia

3. The priority treatment is vagal maneuvers and intravenous (IV) administration of 6 mg of adenosine followed by 12 mg of adenosine if first dose is not effective.
4. He is now unstable; immediate cardioversion at 50 to 100 J is required (consider sedation).
5. Normal sinus rhythm
6. Caffeine, fatigue, stress, and dehydration

Test Yourself!

1. d
2. c
3. c
4. a
5. b

Practice Strips

2.1 sinus bradycardia with depressed ST segments

2.2 normal sinus rhythm

2.3 normal sinus rhythm

2.4 sinus tachycardia

2.5 sinus arrhythmia

Chapter 3

Case Study

1. The immediate priority intervention is to assess the pulse; if there is no pulse, start chest compressions at a rate of at least 100 beats/minute and a ratio of 30 compressions to two breaths (30:2).
2. Ventricular fibrillation
3. Defibrillation
4. The first drug administered is epinephrine 1-mg IV, after the second defibrillation.
5. The immediate priority intervention is to assess blood pressure (B/P), airway, level of consciousness, and continue to monitor the rhythm closely.

Test Yourself!

1. Ventricular fibrillation/pulseless ventricular tachycardia

2. a. D
   b. D
   c. C
   d. D

3. a. Unifocal
   b. Multifocal
   c. Couplets
   d. Bigeminy

4. a. True

5. Epinephrine 1-mg IV bolus

Practice Strips

3.1 sinus rhythm with premature junctional contraction (PJC) (5th beat)

3.2 junctional rhythm

3.3 junctional rhythm with inverted T waves

3.4 accelerated junctional rhythm

3.5 junctional tachycardia

3.6 sinus tachycardia with one premature ventricular contraction (PVC)

3.7 sinus rhythm with bigeminal PVCs

3.8 sinus rhythm with multifocal PVCs

3.9 ventricular tachycardia (11 beats)

3.10 ventricular tachycardia

3.11 ventricular fibrillation

3.12 aganol rhythm

3.13 accelerated idioventricular rhythm

3.14 idioventricular rhythm

Chapter 4

Case Study

1. Second-degree AV block Type II

2. Unstable (B/P decreased, level of consciousness decreased)

3. The required priority treatments are 12-lead EKG, oxygen by nasal cannula, pacing, or a vasopressor infusion (i.e., dopamine or epinephrine).

4. No

5. The potential causes of this rhythm are inferior MI, anterior MI, or ischemia.

Test Yourself!

1. a

2. The PR interval progressively gets longer until a beat is dropped.

3. a. True

4. The two AV blocks that do not require urgent treatment are first-degree AV block and second-degree Type I (Wenkebach).

5. In third-degree heart block, there is no relationship between the P waves and the QRS. Therefore, the P–P is regular and the R–R is regular.

Practice Strips

4.1 sinus rhythm with first-degree AV block

4.2 second-degree AV block Type I

4.3 second-degree AV block Type II

Chapter 5

Case Study

1. Sinus bradycardia

2. The rhythm on the strip indicates failure to capture.

3. The priority treatment includes turning up the milliamperes (mA) and checking the battery assessing the patient (A,B,C) and calling for help, this is an emergency.

4. A potential alternative would be permanent pacemaker insertion.

5. The complications the patient must be observed for are hemorrhage, air embolus, pneumothorax, arrhythmias, hematoma, perforation of the right ventricle.

Test Yourself!

1. c

2. For potential causes of pulseless electrical activity, see Table 5.1.

3. a

4. b

Practice Strips

5.1 100% ventricular paced, no intrisic rhythm, no malfunction

5.2 atrial paced, failure to sense, underlying rhythm third-degree heart block

5.3 ventricular paced, failure to capture, no intrinsic rhythm

5.4 ventricular paced, failure to sense, underlying sinus bradycardia rhythm

Chapter 6

Case Study

1. Inferior myocardial infarction

Test Yourself!

1. b

2. c

3. b

4. a

Chapter 7

Case Study

1. The priority actions are to assess circulation, airway, and breathing, if no pulse, start cardiopulmonary resuscitation (CPR) immediately and activate a code blue (cardiac arrest).

2. Torsades de pointes
3. This rhythm occurred because of hypomagnesemia caused by prolonged diarrhea.

Test Yourself!

1. The risk of a prolonged QT interval is the R-on-T phenomenon, which can lead to ventricular fibrillation.
2. On an EKG, hyperkalemia = tall, peaked T waves, whereas hypokalemia = flattened T waves with possible emergence of a U wave immediately following the T wave.
3. c
4. a

Index